BEYOND MAINTENANCE

Papers from a Drug Treatment Seminar
organised by
the Irish Catholic Bishops' Conference
in association with *The Irish Times*

Edited by Bishop Eamonn Walsh

VERITAS

Published 2000 by
Veritas Publications
7/8 Lower Abbey Street
Dublin 1

ISBN 1 85390 512 7

British Library Cataloguing
in Publication Data.
A catalogue record for
this book is available
from the British Library.

Cover design by Bill Bolger
Printed in the Republic of Ireland by Betaprint Ltd, Dublin

CONTENTS

INTRODUCTION

The papers published in this book capture the context and content of the 'Beyond Maintenance' Seminar organised by the Bishops' Drugs Initiative Committee in association with *The Irish Times*.

At the time of its establishment in 1997, the Bishops' Drugs Initiative made a conscious decision to concentrate on 'street drugs' rather than on alcohol or prescribed medicines. The Initiative was to be another shoulder to the wheel of the existing voluntary and statutory bodies in the area of drug treatment and prevention rather than re-inventing the wheel.

The Church has an access to people who might not be as readily available to other bodies. This access is a valuable resource that can be used to encourage those who are suffering to seek help; to educate people towards prevention; to encourage all the community to support those in need of help; to report back on what is working or not working and to highlight existing and emerging needs.

The Church can help in many ways to introduce drug education programmes into schools and to ensure that these are of high quality. Priests, Sisters and Brothers are members or Chairpersons of many School Boards of Management, especially in the primary education sector; members of Religious Orders are responsible for many schools; Diocesan Advisors have responsibility for overseeing the teaching of religious education in schools. Lay people who are members of the Church play even more important roles as teachers and as parents.

The Church, through her members who are involved in varied works and disciplines, also has a contribution to make in teasing out what constitutes good policy and practice for drug treatment, prevention and education.

The Bishops' Network of Contact Persons comprises social workers, gardaí, health board staff, clergy, religious, counsellors and other disciplines, with one or two people representing each diocese. The Contact Persons find that working in regions rather than nationally is both more effective and convenient. The regions are

Killarney, Sligo, Derry and Dublin, based on the four provinces of the Bishops' Conference. In recent months, some of the Health Boards have expressed an active interest in working more closely with the Contact Persons at local and diocesan levels.

Through the advice of the Bishops' network of Contact Persons in the twenty-six dioceses, which include the thirty-two counties, the Bishops' Drugs Initiative established priorities. *Breaking the Silence* was published in 1997 in an effort to assure those misusing drugs and their families that there is no need to suffer in silence; it helps to talk and help is available. In 1998 the clear message was that no one person, no statutory or voluntary body, can successfully address the drugs issues without community support. This resulted in the publication of *Tackling Drug Problems Together.*

The community groups, during 1999 and 2000, especially in the Limerick and Dublin regions, kept emphasising the need for holistic treatment that would address all the problems and issues that may underline or accompany drug misuse. In 1999 the Bishops' Drugs Initiative invited the Irish Centre for Faith and Culture to address 'A Faith Response to the Street Drug Culture'. They examined the faith and spirituality at play in the lives of drug users and the spiritual component of drug treatment programmes.

It is quite evident from the Report that there is a spiritual hunger among those who use drugs and a desire among the vast majority of Centres to have a spiritual component that is adaptable to individual needs. The *Beyond Maintenance* Seminar was an attempt to address all of the needs of drug-users. The Bishops' Drugs Initiative Team is most grateful to Minister Eoin Ryan for his support of the Seminar through his Address, presence and participation in the Question and Answer session. He highlighted the positive contribution that a spiritual programme can make to those in recovery. Other speakers and the participants endorsed this point during the Questions and Answers session. The Faith and Culture Working Party kindly agreed to the inclusion of their Report in this book because of its relevance to the holistic care and treatment of those affected by drug misuse.

The Editor of *The Irish Times,* Mr Conor Brady, readily agreed to co-sponsor the seminar when approached. He emphasised that as a national daily newspaper they wished to encourage debate that would heighten public awareness of the extent and nature of Ireland's drug problems. 'I believe it is absolutely crucial to highlight drug abuse. It is an issue that has far-reaching effects on the daily lives of the community, and public awareness is essential.' The support of *The Irish Times* has been central to the success of the seminar.

I wish to thank all who contributed to this publication, which contains hard facts, heart-rending testimonies, recommendations based on research, and the experience of varied disciplines working with those affected by drug misuse. Special thanks to Paula O'Gorman of *The Irish Times*, Chris Murphy and Susan O'Neill of the Drugs Awareness Programme, Crosscare, Father Paul Lavelle and Peter O'Brien, and to all members of the Seminar Organising Committee.

Finally, I would like to thank the staff of Veritas, particularly Maura Hyland, Colette Dower and Aideen Quigley, for their help in publishing these papers.

✠ *Bishop Eamonn Walsh*
Chairperson, Bishops' Drugs Initiative Committee

OPENING ADDRESS

Archbishop Desmond Connell

I welcome you all who have taken the time to attend and participate in this Seminar. I extend a warm welcome to Ms Jane Wilson and Dr Des Corrigan, our main speakers today, and to Mr Eoin Ryan TD, Minister of State for Local Development with special responsibility for National Drugs Strategy, who will address this Seminar this afternoon.

As members of Voluntary Statutory Bodies, as families, friends and concerned people, we are all anxious to do what is best in the battle against drugs and their misuse. I welcome you all.

This Jubilee Year Seminar, which is being organised by the Bishops' Drugs Initiative Committee in association with *The Irish Times,* is very timely. It comes at a time when the Government is reviewing the National Drugs Strategy. The tragic reality of drug deaths has been vividly put before us in recent weeks.

As was stated in the Pastoral Letter of the Bishops' Conference in 1997, *Breaking the Silence,* we welcome programmes that help people with drug problems to establish greater stability in their lives and ideally to withdraw from all drugs. We are challenged here today to discuss ways of approaching development, such as an extension of counselling programmes, so that those on methadone maintenance can live a life free of drugs. Recognition of drug use and drug problems, and subsequent intervention, involve knowledge and skills, which can be shared at a Seminar like this one today. Methadone maintenance was originally intended as a temporary measure but is by definition long-term. We must challenge users to cease using drugs and lead them to a drug-free lifestyle. Part of our objective is to identify behavioural therapies and counselling, together with other supportive services, to assist drug users and their families.

It should be recognised that the authorities have greatly improved treatment programmes in recent years. Nonetheless, it is estimated that in the Dublin area alone, more than four hundred heroin users are waiting to join treatment programmes. Opiate abuse has been largely a Dublin problem, but there is evidence recently that it is emerging in other towns and cities. This has been confirmed to the Bishops' Drugs Initiative Committee by the Contact Persons in each diocese.

It has also become clear that the way forward is for Contact Persons to work primarily on a regional basis, focusing on area needs. The regions are co-ordinated by Bishop Murphy in Killarney, Bishop Jones in Sligo, Bishop Lagan in Derry, Bishop Ó Ceallaigh and Bishop Walsh in Dublin.

From the outset, the Bishops' Drugs Initiative pledged to work in close cooperation with the local and national voluntary and statutory bodies and to play our part through the unique contacts the Church has with her people. The Church is one voice among many who are trying to give hope and help to those affected directly and indirectly by drug misuse.

Perhaps I should add that, just as there are two aspects of the problem of poverty and privation – a) immediate need to which we respond with appropriate assistance, and b) reflection upon the disorders within our society that create problems of poverty and destitution, so likewise there are two aspects of the problem of drug-taking – a) the immediate needs of those who are in the grip of addiction, and b) reflection on the deeper causes that lead young people in particular to succumb to drug-taking. Our seminar today is concerned with the first of these two aspects but I would wish to say, in the presence of the media, that we have great need of the reflection that will enable us to address the deeper causes of drug-taking. Why are so many, particularly young people, bored in circumstances more affluent than obtained even in the recent past? What is the connection between boredom and drug-taking? No doubt there are many different sociological, psychological and philosophical ways of approaching this matter. The Church has a uniquely profound contribution to make, and it has need of the support that is so evident today in the participation of *The Irish Times* in our seminar as it seeks to address the question.

I ask God's blessing on this seminar and all who, with its assistance, may be influenced for the good.

NATIONAL EXTENT OF THE DRUG PROBLEM IN IRELAND

Jim Cusack

In looking into the extent of the drug problem in Ireland, I have examined some statistics from Garda and RUC files on drugs cases from 1979 onwards. The figures are striking in one respect. There is an inexorable increase in seizures and arrests. Year on year in both jurisdictions, the amounts of both Class A drugs (such as heroin, cocaine, crack, ecstasy and hallucinogenics) and Class B drugs (such as cannabis and speed) increases.

The figures are like something out a Soviet Five-Year Plan. There were 5,924 arrests for drug offences in 1998 – five times more than 1993 and ten times more than 1978.

In 1998, 600,000 ecstasy tablets were seized compared to only 429 in 1991. We are importing tons of cannabis each year, whereas there were only a few stone coming in twenty years ago. Cocaine, formerly the expensive drug of preference among our social elite, is now flooding into the country by the sackload. About a metric ton of cocaine has been seized by the Gardaí in the past five years. The Gardaí have made almost 60,000 charges for the 'misuse' of drugs in twenty years.

Heroin remains our most damaging illegal drug. Crack cocaine has not caught on here, though cocaine-cocktail use by heroin addicts is becoming a significant feature of abuse in this city. Until the late 1980s and early 1990s, seizures of heroin in the Republic were measured annually in grams. The seizure figures are now measured in kilos. The last available figures here, for 1998, show that the Gardaí seized thirty-eight kilos of heroin. In 1988 the figure was less than half a kilo. Some seventy kilos of heroin were seized between 1993 and 1998 in this State. In the previous decade, in the years between 1983 and 1988, the total was only 5.5 kilos.

These figures tend to support the reports from health and social agencies that the addict population of Dublin has increased dramatically in the same period. It is estimated at around 15,000 now, whereas I recollect that, only a few years ago, there was a general belief that it was less than half that number. I mention Dublin rather than the rest of the country here, because Garda statistics also tend to support the belief that the Republic's heroin problem is concentrated in the city. Some 99 per cent of heroin seizures and arrests are in Dublin. The concentrations of Garda heroin seizures and arrests are still in the traditional working-class centres, where the drug made its original impact in the late 1970s and 1980s.

From a media perspective, heroin is still treated here as a part of the wider crime problem. The orthodoxy is that it is a 'scourge' that must be wiped out, somehow, through mainly traditional policing and through the application of punishment or reform of the addict through prison and probation.

The rising tide of heroin and other drugs in this country is not a favourite theme in speeches by politicians and Garda leaders. Government and senior members of the Gardaí concentrate more on improving crime figures. After two decades of rising crime, the police and politicians are enjoying the fourth consecutive year of reduced crime figures. There has been a noticeable reduction in crime in this State. But this is in line with the improvements in the economy, providing job prospects for young men who might otherwise be on the streets.

The very real scourge of heroin-related crime that Dublin witnessed in the 1970s and 1980s, with dozens of robberies and muggings each day, has died away. The price of heroin has fallen dramatically in the past decade. There isn't the same economic necessity for addicts to rob as there was ten years ago.

Methadone has almost certainly played a major contributory role. People are much less likely to commit crime when they are on methadone stabilisation. There may also be a correlation here between the introduction of methadone treatment and the price reduction in heroin. Suppliers, seeing their addict market being reduced by a stabilising alternative, have to react. The most obvious way is to make the product more attractive by decreasing its price.

And this dramatic price reduction is possible because there is a world glut of heroin. State Department figures show the US market for heroin has stopped growing but production has increased in Southern and Central American, eastern European, western African and Asian countries.

Europol, the EU's infant criminal intelligence agency, reports that organised crime gangs from as many as thirty-seven different countries are now in competition to supply the European market with drugs. The Turkish gangs, with both left- and right-wing political connections in their own country, have dominated the heroin supply routes until now. There is now much more competition and, unless the international criminal gangs can agree a cartel, it is likely the price of heroin will remain low for the foreseeable future. Given these global movements and market forces, it would seem likely that heroin importation will continue to increase in the Republic and Northern Ireland and there will be more addiction.

I believe, to a certain extent, that our thinking on drug problems here has tended to be parochial. We are merely a small offshore market for a tremendously well-organised global trade. The greatest power in the history of the world, the United States, has been fighting in vain to reduce global heroin supply for over twenty years without success.

One of our nearest EU neighbours, the Netherlands, with the largest seaport in the world, is now one of the biggest, if not the biggest clearing-house for the international drugs trade. It is no surprise that our organised criminals, faced with assets seizure at home, have merely moved to the source of their supply, which is within commuting distance of Dublin.

As I have said, heroin does not appear to be showing any great deal of movement out of the city – yet. But there is a worrying increase in the amount of drug abuse outside Dublin. Areas where, until quite recently, there were almost no recreational drugs among young people, are now reported by Gardaí to be awash with cannabis and ecstasy. The Garda figures for drug seizures and arrests show dramatic increases in every rural division. This is not due to Gardaí outside of Dublin paying more attention to drugs, rather, it is because there are more drugs than ever before in the rest of the country. The figures may still be relatively small, but ten-fold increases in drug seizures in rural divisions in the past decade are not unusual. If this continues, the rest of the country will have begin to have a problem. If the recreational Class B abuse continues in rural Ireland as it is doing, it may only be a matter of time before the Class A drugs arrive.

The North is experiencing a near identical boom in the use of recreational, or Class B, drugs. Ecstasy seizures by the RUC in the 1990s often outstripped seizures here. Cocaine abuse in the North has increased dramatically. A small but growing heroin problem has been developing in the housing estates of southeast Antrim in the past decade, and it is now taking hold in towns like Ballymena and Antrim. Some of the housing estates around these two towns are now suffering the same sort of plight that Dublin estates suffered in the 1970s. As with Dublin thirty years ago, there is widespread ignorance in the North about heroin addiction and very few resources for addicts.

Belfast is an obvious next target for the heroin trade but, for the moment, the Loyalist paramilitary figures that dominate the drugs trade in the North are holding back from involvement in heroin because of its perceived anti-social connotations. The paramilitaries depend on the community support for survival. If they are seen selling heroin, they leave themselves open to rejection. However, heroin is creeping into Protestant working-class areas. There are signs that ex-Republican paramilitaries are providing protection for drug dealers in Catholic areas.

One of the possible dangerous future trends – and there is evidence that this has begun – is the movement of former paramilitaries into the drugs trade. They will bring their specialisations in professional violence to the trade. Many are expert in smuggling and have contacts abroad in the arms trade. It is not a short step from guerrilla warfare to organised crime, but it is a path that has been taken by others including the Italian Mafia and the Chinese Triads.

FAMILY EXPERIENCES OF DRUG MISUSE AND THE ROAD TO RECOVERY

A Son and Mother

A Son's Testimony

From an addict's point of view, I had faced many difficulties when I eventually decided it was time to try and stop using. Without blaming the system, I know it all fell back to me as a person and how badly I wanted to stop using. But as many addicts would feel, I felt like there was no hope, I was down and out and the world was against me.

This was just the way my life was meant to be, but I didn't want it anymore. I thought I was just a junkie who didn't believe in himself, nor did anyone else. I had tried many things over the years in order to get clean and stay clean. I had tried staying at home and doing it on my own, going through my sickness with my head racing and contemplating suicide many times, only to get six or seven days clean and thinking, 'nice one, I have cracked it, I'm free,' and swearing to myself and pleading with God never to let me end up where I had just finished. But to my despair I'd only find myself ending up even worse within days and thinking, 'what do I have to do to beat this?'

So I went on to try many detox's and found not one to work and then I ended up on maintenance for three years and also using at the same time, plus still wanting to get clean, but the flame that I had left in my spirit was slowly burning itself out. The pain I felt was unimaginable to some, and so was the dark place in my head. My heart felt like a truck had run over it many times. On the outside I looked like I had just pulled myself out of the gutter – I was a mere six and a half stone. In my time of using I had hit many a rock-bottom, but this one felt different. I knew it was either do or die.

At this stage I had more of a will to die than I had to live, as the way I had been living was not good enough. I would think to myself if this is what life is about I don't want it. So in my heart I began to lie down and die.

So I think, 'right this is it, I am going to give it my best shot, and if it doesn't work I will end it.' So I began to look for help. I tried many places for many days, not only ringing but presenting myself at their doors, only to be rejected time and time again.

At this stage there was very little spirit left in me. Every hour seemed like a day and it was harder and harder to hang on. So I rang Sr Consilio's [Cuan Mhuire in Bruree, Co Limerick, one of the Cuan Mhuire centres founded by Sr Consilio] and told them I was an alcoholic and they agreed to see me in two weeks. While waiting I tried many other places only to be turned away for one reason or another, and as time went by I was getting closer to death's door. In those three weeks I spent each day wishing I was dead.

I would be in the house sticking needles in myself and I would cry because I didn't want to do it, but not knowing how not to do it was the problem. At one stage I fell to my knees and cried, 'Oh Jesus Christ, please take me out of this, I can't take it anymore'. Eventually the time came and I went into treatment and I cried like a child would for his soother, why I don't know. I spent six months there under the care of very understanding and caring people, who helped me more than anyone could imagine. God knows I needed it and most importantly I got it.

Today I am five years clean and sober and the better for it. I am now trying to make a difference for the still-suffering addict.

Out of all those times of trying, all it would have taken was for someone to treat me like a human being. It didn't take other drugs or doctors, all it took was a small bit of love. And compassion, it goes a long way – the bit I got is still going and I will try to pass it on.

With my greatest appreciation to those who cared for me, Nurse Jim, Christy, Gerry, Sean, Declan, Nurse Ellen, Nurse Ann, Nurse Liz, Nurse Kathleen, Sr Consilio and Sr Agnes.

A Mother's Testimony

In May 1995, after realising that maybe this time my son was actually serious about going into a treatment centre, I was panic-stricken: 'Where do I go? Who do I see?' These were the first questions that I asked myself. I knew of a methadone clinic in the city centre because my son had told me about it.

I went in with my son and was turned away by a receptionist, because I had no appointment. I knew if my son was not given any help now I would probably find him dead. And I broke down. At this stage they sent for a counsellor to see me who gave me an appointment for two weeks later for myself and not for my son (which, by the way, she was later to cancel). I refused to leave until I got one for my son and so they gave me one for four weeks later.

After these heartbreaking four weeks, we returned to the clinic yet again. They assessed him and put him on a waiting list and we were once again sent home. Two days after this a friend of my son's called to my home and told me that my son was going to kill himself. I hysterically went to a man who I knew helped addicts in the area, and who was himself a recovering addict.

He brought me to see many people, too numerous to mention, and again and again my hopes were shattered when we were turned away. I couldn't bear the thought of any more doors closing on me, because every day my son was getting closer to death.

He then gave me the phone number of a sister who ran a treatment centre in Limerick. He told me to say that my son was an alcoholic and not to mention his drug addiction until he was in the door. After speaking to Sister Agnes on the phone, she told me to bring him to see her in Bruree in two weeks' time with his clothes. She also told me that this did not mean that he would be taken in.

For the next two weeks we bought methadone on the streets and detoxed him at home (or so we thought). We then brought him to Limerick, where he was welcomed with open arms and they loved him and showed him how to love himself again. From that day to this my son has been clean and sober and recovering every day, as he says, one day at a time.

For the angels of Bruree, because I believe that that is what they truly are, I will always be grateful, and words could never express my gratitude.

I have my son back.

POSITIVE AND NEGATIVE EXPERIENCES OF COMMUNITIES THAT HAVE SUFFERED THE DRUGS PROBLEM IN DUBLIN

Anna Quigley

Background and History

The background and history of the drugs problem in Dublin over the last twenty-five years and how this has been handled gives us some insight into the situation of communities that have suffered the drug problem in Dublin, and how they have been affected. There has been a huge neglect of Dublin's drug problem, particularly the heroin problem, over the past twenty-five years. That fact is no longer disputed.

In 1982 the Bradshaw report was published into abuse in the North inner city. It showed that there was a higher rate of heroin abuse in that area than in those parts of New York that were notorious for having a severe drug problem. It showed that 10 per cent of the 15-24 age group were using heroin. This research was undertaken by the government at the time in an attempt to disprove claims by community activists of a serious drug problem.

The National Co-ordinating Committee on Drug Abuse was established in response to the Bradshaw Report in 1983 and they identified at that time what was identified again thirteen years later by the 1996 Task Force – a serious heroin problem in areas of Dublin that were marginalised and disadvantaged. They recommended a huge programme of investment in community and youth structures. Their report was never published.

Through the rest of the 1980s and 1990s the problem spread to all the other marginalised and disadvantaged areas of the city. We therefore cannot say that there was a lack of knowledge, that nobody knew of the drug problem. Action could have been taken as far back as 1982-83. There is still a sense in local communities that they were abandoned, and that will take a long time to change or forget.

Since the 1996 Ministerial Task Force report (the one that was acted upon), a lot has happened. National and local Task Forces were set up and there has been a huge expansion in services. In the Eastern Regional Health Authority area alone, there were 1,000 people in drug treatment in 1996. This year there are approximately 4,500. There have been many changes also in the area of drug crime legislation. However, we are still playing catch-up. We are clearly not on top of the problem because you cannot make up for twenty-five years of neglect in three or four years.

Positive Experiences

A large level of community involvement: This positive comes from the experienced 'negative' of pure desperation. Communities found no help or support from the State and they had to get directly involved. People started out by lobbying and campaigning for treatment and counselling services, especially the parents and families of addicts. This community involvement cannot in any way be taken for granted and needs continuous support and resourcing.

Involvement of local task forces: For the first time, communities have been given a role in drawing up plans for the allocation of resources in their own areas and there has been a formal recognition that the communities have played a leading role in this issue.

Networking: Different communities have greatly benefitted from networking, which enables them to provide support to each other, share their collected knowledge and wisdom, and have an effective input into policy making. The Dublin CityWide Drugs Crisis Campaign grew out of this and there has been an ongoing partnership between all the agencies and community groups involved.

Family support groups: These grew mainly out of a sense of isolation, of not knowing where to turn for help. They held the service of commemoration and hope in Sean McDermott Street Church last February as a public recognition of the grief and suffering of these people over the past twenty years. If a similar number of young people in our country had died from any other cause, there would have been a national outcry. But because it was from drug abuse, they were seen in some way to be undeserving of real action. These families can also have a say in how drug treatment services develop and can continue to ask for support services for families of addicts.

A major expansion in services in recent years. There are as many as 220 funded local projects, some for rehabilitation and some for prevention.

Negative experiences

Some communities' reactions: Some people in communities want drug rehabilitation services in their own areas; but others have the opposite reaction. The latter may be a form of denial: 'We don't have this problem here.' There may even be a tinge of snobbery to it. This has led to feelings of both isolation and fear – isolation caused by other people judging those who have a family member with a problem and the shame and the guilt that follows from it, and fear caused by the image that some people have of drug dealers, users and pushers.

Sometimes it's easier to stay silent. The bishops' use of the phrase 'breaking the silence' from 1997 is very relevant. This silence can add weight to the view that communities don't need services in their own area.

A second negative reaction comes from people looking for an easy solution. It grows out of the notion that if you identify the person, then you identify the problem, and if you get rid of the person, then you get rid of the problem. Some community responses have been about just that: getting people out of their area and moving them on. You can understand how people might want a quick and simple solution to a drug problem in their area. All of us are afraid of things we don't understand. But at the same time, these perceptions must be challenged. People need to be informed. Discussion needs to take place and communities must not be allowed to give in to the fear and the silence.

Leadership in this regard has been sorely lacking from some politicians and the Church. The challenge for the Church is to provide support mechanisms for priests so that they are properly informed about what services need to be provided, and what they can do to help communities in their care.

The media can be less than helpful in the language they use in their portrayal of drug users. Stereotypes do not help informed discussion. They only add to the prejudice and hysteria.

The 'Catch-up Syndrome': Services have been developed in response to a crisis. We have not had the luxury of planning them properly. People now have a greater understanding that treatment is not just about the medical aspect. They were once grateful just to have clinics. Now they understand that drug abuse is not a medical problem. It is a problem that has a medical aspect. The whole range of support services – counselling, family support, therapies, aftercare, rehabilitation, relapse and respite care – this is what we mean by treatment. The medical aspect alone will not work without other aspects of support also being in place.

The 'methadone vs. drug free' debate is a waste of time and a distraction. It is not helpful to set one up against the other as a simplistic for or against situation. Different options will work for different people. It is more important to concentrate on putting in place a broad range of treatments that work. For some users, treatment may include methadone, for others it may not. The key issue around methadone remains the overall context in which it is used. Our services at present, however, are extremely inadequate because services developed in a crisis situation do not develop in an ideal way.

The tip of the iceberg: People look at the amount of money being spent on the drug problem and only see it getting worse. Of course it is only when you address the underlying issues that you can truly ascertain the actual level of need. When you start to put services in place for addicts, you discover the need for family support, which further leads you to the need for child care. Every issue addressed raises further issues and a deeper level of need becomes apparent.

According to Catherine Cumiskey's report, *Estimating the Prevalence of Opiate Drug Use in Dublin, Ireland, During 1996,* 'Using all three data sources [the central methadone patient treatment list, the hospital in-patient inquiry database (HIPE), and the Garda Siochána database] it was estimated that there were 13,460 opiate users in Dublin in 1996.' The current figure for those in drug treatment, according to the Eastern Health Board, is 4,500. Therefore we can say that there are approximately 10,000 users not in touch with the services now provided. This puts community groups in a difficult position, as they had believed that if these services were provided, the situation would improve.

The situation has improved for those who have availed of these services. But for the communities themselves, sometimes things do not get better. Many have not yet been helped, and the underlying causes of drug addiction have not yet been addressed.

The broader context: There is a sense that the drug problem will be solved if the gardaí get enough resources and seize enough kilos of drugs, and if enough services are provided. That shows a lack of understanding of the drug problem and why it persists in our society. Every Government department must realise that they have a part to play in eliminating the underlying causes of the drug problem. We have not yet reached the stage where everyone can see how our drug problem is linked into how our society is structured and how we live as a society. Until the underlying causes of the drug problem are addressed, the problem will continue.

SUBSTANCE MISUSE
IN THE NEW MILLENNIUM

Jane Wilson

Introduction

The last few decades have witnessed an explosion of drug misuse amongst young people. In the early '80s heroin was introduced into socially disadvantaged areas in major cities right across Europe. The impact was devastating, and resulted in the emergence of a new, highly dependent, predominantly drug-injecting population.

Within a few years this growing drug epidemic held within it the seeds of a potential HIV epidemic. The discovery that many of these young heroin users had contracted the HIV virus created shock waves in society. Defined as a population of young, highly mobile and sexually active injectors, they were considered a particularly high-risk group for both contracting and spreading the virus.

A rapid and effective response was required, and by the end of the '80s the development of harm reduction strategies, which included needle exchanges and prescribing, was well under way. Understandably, there was resistance to these policies from some sectors in the field. However, it was primarily the need to contain the HIV epidemic as a public health priority that underpinned the setting up of these new services.

In recent years, awareness of the medical problems in this group has been eclipsed by accumulating evidence that they also have more serious mental health problems that had not been previously recognised. The rates of dual diagnosis (the co-existence of a mental health problem and a substance misuse problem) are strikingly high amongst drug users. The additional problems associated with a dual diagnosis have recently become the focus of intense investigation and we have recently been made aware of the additional difficulties that this diagnosis carries.

Parallel to this, research emanating from the trauma field has shown that those who have experienced childhood abuse and neglect are at high risk of developing both psychological and substance misuse problems in adulthood. Not surprisingly, there is now robust evidence that indicates that a very high proportion of those with a dual diagnosis will also have a history of child abuse.

We are coming to realise that an overwhelming number of our young drug users have more than 'double trouble'. They are characterised as having considerable biopsychosocial issues to contend with. The multiplicity, severity and chronicity of these problems are seen to create a matrix of disadvantage within which substance misuse plays a part but is not the only issue.

The landscape has altered dramatically in the last decade. We now better understand the nature and characteristics of this group. Studies show that they have more psychiatric problems, increased medical problems, more criminal involvement and more difficulties with family and social relationships. The impact of these multiple problems on treatment utilisation, not just within the addiction field but across all public health and social welfare sectors, is of growing concern.

We are faced with tremendous challenges and today's seminar is a timely response to these challenges. The complexity of issues involved may require not only consideration of what options exist 'beyond maintenance' but also how we can enhance existing services and introduce new systems of support that can adequately respond to these problems. Today we have a unique opportunity to contribute our knowledge, creativity, compassion and vision in an effort to achieve this goal.

Mental Health and Substance Misuse

Many of those working with drug users have increasingly voiced concern about the rising numbers of users who present at services with considerable mental health problems alongside their substance misuse problems (Wilson 1997).

This concern is mirrored in the rapid growth of literature on the subject. The study and treatment of dual diagnosis in such countries as the USA, Canada, and Australia is quite advanced. However, in recent years there has been a dramatic increase in European research and these studies are now making a considerable contribution to the current pool of knowledge (Hendricks 1990; Kokkevi et al. 1998; Krausz et al. 1998; Ravdnal and Vaglum 1995; Scott and Farrell 1998).

Estimates of substance misuse and psychiatric co-morbidity have been drawn from various types of investigations across a range of populations, which include community and general population surveys as well as studies on incarcerated and treatment populations. High rates of co-ocurrence have been found across these groups. The Epidemiologic Catchment Area (ETA) was one of the first projects to document such high rates of co-occurence in a survey of more than 20,000 people in five areas in the USA (Regier et al. 1990).

Significant findings include the following: an additional DSM-III-R mental disorder was diagnosed in more than half the drug abusers (53%); the relative risk of drug abusers suffering from an additional mental disorder was 4.5 times higher than for all other participants in the study; the rates for drug abusers in treatment were even higher, with 64% meeting criteria for a coexisting mental disorder and 37% of those with an alcohol abuse or dependence disorder met criteria for a mental disorder other than drug abuse or dependence.

The National Co-morbidity Survey (NCS) in Great Britain surveyed over 1000 people in the community and in institutionalised populations. They reported that 58% of all current disorders and 88% of severe current disorders were found among the 13% of the population with a lifetime history of dual diagnosis (Kessler et al. 1997).

In research on substance-abuse populations, a Dutch study of methadone maintenance clients found that 41% were diagnosed with a major psychiatric disorder and 35% of the remaining group were diagnosed as having personality disorders. In only 20% of the sample could no diagnosis be made (Derks 1990). In a recent German study on a similar population, psychiatric disorders were established for 55% of the participants (Ravdnal and Vaglum 1995).

Studies on psychiatric in-patient populations ratify the high incidence of substance misuse among this population (Mueser 1992; Appleby et al. 1997), as do those in emergency departments (Barbee et al. 1989). One study reported that 78% of those assessed at psychiatric units reported lifetime incidence of drug or alcohol misuse

(Kulka et al. 1990). A study of young chronic patients at a community mental health centre found that 44% were currently using drugs and 29% had used drugs in the past (Safer 1987).

However, the problem of dual diagnosis is wider than the mental health and addiction fields. If you examine prevalence in other areas, such as the criminal justice system and the homeless, field rates of substance misuse and psychiatric disorders appear highest in these populations.

The highest rates of dual diagnosis were found in the prison population. The ETA study estimated that 90% of inmates surveyed in prison who had a mental disorder also had a substance misuse disorder (Regier et al. 1990). Other research found that 25% of addicted offenders had a lifetime history of major depression and bipolar disorder and 9% had a history of schizophrenia (Chiles et al. 1990). Another study found that 44% of inmates had a lifetime history of substance misuse disorders coexisting with depressive or antisocial personality disorders (Abram and Teplin 1991).

Lastly, a study on homeless patients entering substance misuse treatment revealed that 60% of the participants had one or more serious mental illness. 38% were diagnosed with major depression, 34% with schizophrenia and 13% with mania. When other mental disorders such as post-traumatic stress disorder and phobia were included, 82% of the patients had diagnoses of serious mental illness as well as a substance misuse disorder (Sacks and De Leon 1997).

Disturbingly, findings consistently reveal that drug users with mental health issues have poorer outcomes in treatment and increased severity of problems than those without mental health issues. In reviewing the research, there is robust evidence that demonstrates that they exhibit poor compliance with prescribing regimes and make excessive use of emergency services (Drake and Brunett 1998; Brown, Stout and Mueller 1996; Osher and Kofoed 1989). Rates of relapse, readmission and hospitalisation are much higher where co-morbidity exists (Coryell, Endicott and Winokur 1992; Bartles et al. 1991).

Housing instability and homelessness is also characteristic of those with a dual diagnosis (Johnson 1997). A number of studies have found that they have elevated rates of violent and criminal behaviour

(Wallace et al. 1998; Jemelka, Trupin and Chiles 1989). They have been found to be at increased risk of HIV infection (Zierler et al. 1991); are associated with increased levels of family stress and dysfunction, and have considerably increased rates of suicide and deliberate self-harm (Wilson 1997; Lucks 1997).

By the early 1990s it was becoming clear that existing treatment provision of all kinds was failing this population. Their interactive symptomatology had a synergistic effect that seemed to create a downward spiral in all areas of functioning (Dansky et al. 1995).

Trauma and Dual Diagnosis – The Connection
It had always been acknowledged that the childhood histories of many addicts were characterised by abuse and neglect and that their life histories continued to reflect high levels of traumatic experiences. What was less well understood at that time was the extent of trauma produced by these experiences and the severity of problems across behavioural, interpersonal, physical, psychological and social domains that could result.

What we do know from treatment outcome evaluation is that family involvement and family support for drug users is a significant factor in their success. While some drug users have this support there are unfortunately many who do not and whose families are also struggling with many social, psychological and addiction issues. In such situations there is a higher risk of child abuse and neglect, which can have a considerable impact on adult functioning and is highly associated with substance misuse in adult life. These entire families need support and intervention and we must consider ways that are not demeaning to engage them in treatment.

The relationship of substance misuse and a history of child abuse has been established in countless studies over the past twenty years.

PREVALENCE OF TRAUMA HISTORIES
IN SUBSTANCE MISUSERS

		F	M
Miller 1987	(A)	67%	
Roshenow 1988		77%	42 %
Yandow 1989	(A)	75%	
Copeland 1992		47%	
Paone 1992		46%	
Miller 1993	(A)	66%	
Fullilove 1993		59%	
Porter 1994		90%	37%
Gil-Rivas 1996		51.2% CSA	12.8%
Brady 1994		73%	
Najavits 1998		85%	

What is striking is not only the high rates of childhood abuse amongst drug users, particularly female drug users, but that these rates are similar to rates for dual diagnosis. Many who are deemed to have a dual diagnosis may well have underlying trauma issues. It it suggested that because the trauma occurred in childhood its impact on development can be more damaging.

IMPACT ON DEVELOPMENT

Like other victims, abused children experience significant psychological distress and dysfunction. Unlike adults, however, they are traumatised during the most critical period of their lives; when assumptions about self, others, and the world are formed; when their relations to their own internal states are being established; and coping and affiliative skills are first acquired.

Such post traumatic reactions can easily have an impact upon subsequent psychological and social maturation, leading to atypical and potentially dysfunctional development. (Briere 1992)

Clearly, childhood abuse is not only the mistreatment of children but can also represent a major lifelong assault on the personhood of the survivor. That this is the case is borne out by the range of long-term effects that are associated with childhood trauma and that operate both intrapsychically and interpersonally. Psychological impairment may include anxiety, low self-esteem, depression, eating disorders, somatic symptoms, self-mutilation, suicidal ideation and substance misuse. Psycho-sexual problems such as aversion to sex, sexual dysfunction, sexual anxiety and guilt, promiscuity and prostitution may develop. Interpersonal difficulties could include distrust, isolation, alienation, fear of others, repeated victimisation in adult relationships, and conflicts in relationships with their children (Bannister 1992).

In light of the potentially damaging long-term sequel, it is not surprising that many survivors would rely on the use of alcohol and drugs as a buffer against the debilitating effects. The use of substances is seen to offer a number of benefits:

> Drugs serve a survivor in numerous ways; they increase the survivor's own tendency to dissociate, they interfere with the memory storage of traumatic experiences, they create some level of well-being, they release inhibitions against expression of painful emotions, rage, sexual expression, and they create social groups that have few demands but in fact may resemble the originally abusive family system. (Trotter 1992)

The self-medication hypothesis is increasingly favoured as a causal explanation of the association between childhood trauma, substance misuse and psychiatric problems (Brown and Wolfe 1994; Stewart 1996). Self-medication can make the 'intolerable' tolerable. Survivors may turn to self-medication to avoid painful memories. These behaviours may be associated with unresolved feelings of conflict, powerlessness and repressed anger and rage resulting from the abuse. This need for 'personal punishment' or 'self-harm' so often noted as a consequence of abuse may represent the ongoing attack on the self due to the shame, guilt and sense of responsibility for the abuse that survivors often feel.

Challenges to Services

The typical profile for those with dual disorders make them system misfits. The range of interconnecting problems they possess extend outside the specific remits of any of the services they are involved with. The assessment and care management systems of each of these services will differ depending on the context within which they identify and respond to problems.

Because they have not been provided with the comprehensive and coordinated services that they require, this group often become 'revolving-door' clients who wander continually between agencies.

They present with complex, interactive symptoms which can elude one-dimensional explanations and treatment approaches. To meet their treatment needs, we must first understand what those needs are. A complete and comprehensive assessment of all potential problem areas may be required if we are to create effective and appropriate packages of care and support.

The contract culture has placed increased pressure on addiction services to demonstrate the efficacy of their practice by improving their monitoring systems and introducing outcome evaluation into their work. These demands for improved documentation have encouraged a reappraisal of assessment protocols in many agencies. Assessment serves multiple purposes, including screening, diagnosis, and treatment planning/outcome evaluation, yet its main purpose must be to create comprehensive care plans and sufficient supports to help drug users move beyond the worlds of pain they often exist in.

These shifts at a policy level dovetail with shifts at the level of service delivery. Many addiction services have expanded their assessment procedures to include some form of mental health screening. However, the addition of mental health assessments may not detect trauma issues that can significantly impede progress.

Yet, while there is increased acceptance of the need to include assessment for mental health problems, there is still considerable resistance to the notion of taking a trauma history. However, many experts in trauma and addiction stress that a trauma history is crucial for developing appropriate care plans and suitable interventions.

ASSESSMENT

The patient profile underscores the need to identify abuse as a critical factor in a patient's history if treatment is to be effective. (Brown, Stout and Mueller 1996)

Implementation of childhood abuse screening instrument significantly increases reporting rates of childhood abuse.... Specific treatment addressing issues related to victimisation might reduce relapse rates among these clients. (Simpson et al. 1994)

Because they seldom volunteer information about their abuse, it is often unreported, undiagnosed and consequently untreated.... Because of the similar defences used to cope with addiction and abuse they may be unable to break the cycle without education and treatment for both problems. A multi modal treatment strategy, utilising interventions for addiction and unresolved trauma, as well as specialised after-care planning appears to be a promising avenue to prepare this group for early abstinence. (Bernstein, Stein and Handelman 1998)

Treatment providers should consider the possibility of a trauma history for any of their revolving-door patients.... If PTSD substance abusers received trauma-specific treatment, they might be less likely to over-utilise or misuse expensive inpatient substance abuse services resulting in substantial clinical care cost savings. (Brown, Stout and Mueller 1996)

Screening for PTSD among women with an addictive disorder should become part of the diagnostic and treatment routine.... As trauma and drug use often covary, it will be difficult, if not impossible, to treat either of these disorders without assessing both. (Fillilove et al. 1993)

The impact of CSA [childhood sexual abuse] on relapse might be influenced by the expertise with which it is addressed in treatment. The severe and complex clinical picture supports recommendations that specialist care be available for CSA survivors in drug and alcohol treatment programs. (Jarvis and Copeland 1997)

Relapse prevention accounts for a major area of work in the addiction field and, as I stressed earlier, failure to assess and address trauma issues may be a hidden factor in the high number of relapses we see in this field.

Treatment Issues

Currently there is an intense debate about types of treatment that should be offered and these are often linked to different philosophical differences and territorial boundaries. Three approaches have been identified as treatment options suitable for drug users with both trauma issues and mental health issues.

The modified substance abuse treatment approach has already begun to be established in this country. Certainly several agencies in Scotland have expanded their assessment procedures, programme content and skills development to better address trauma and mental health issues. Many services are now recruiting staff with a mental health background to compliment existing addiction staff.

Linkage programmes are where comprehensive assessments have been done on clients, and multiple referral and services may be involved in their care. For example, in many drug services, skills for addressing trauma issues are not present and these clients will attend the drug service for their drug problems but also see an abuse counsellor who will work on these issues.

Whereas modified programmes still give primacy to the main presenting problem, integrated programmes are conceptualised, developed and staffed by a team who provided a blended approach to drug users with multiple problems. In several parts of Scotland, dual diagnosis teams and services are beginning to appear in response to the demand by drug services for additional services for this group.

Implementing any of these approaches will require much closer coordination across all sectors involved with drug users. Although programmes to improve liaison between sectors and services may appear attractive, there is concern that a common language for successful communication may not exist. Also there is a body of opinion that argues that integrated treatment, especially for dual diagnosis, must underpin an approach based on assertive community support which would increase collaboration between policy makers, funders, services and the community.

Coordination of services is a crucial element. The following is a list of working principles outlined in a recent report, *Tackling Drugs in Scotland: Action in Partnership* (HMSO 1997):

WORKING PRINCIPLES

Services coordination is usually a slow, evolutionary process.

Services coordination is primarily a consensus-building process.

Organisational changes do not necessarily lead to services coordination.

Successful service coordination depends on the leadership and talents of responsible individuals.

Services coordination may reduce short-term costs but other funding incentives are crucial.

Perception of benefit by service providers from services coordination is crucial.

At the delivery level, effective coordination requires shared information systems.

A common service strategy facilitates services coordination.

Formal inter-organisational agreements facilitate the coordination process.

Being responsible to a common super-ordinate authority facilitates coordination.

Linkages may be likely to be adopted outside major urban areas, but comprehensiveness is difficult to achieve.

Travel times that exceed 45 minutes seem to interfere with coordination between agencies.

Efforts to develop the sharing of an ideology that supports coordination appear worthwhile.

Relevant training and continuing education are necessary for staff dealing with patients, as well as for their supervisors, in a newly coordinated system of services.

This document also outlines ways in which coordination of services can be achieved:

OPTIONS FOR ACHIEVING COORDINATION

Co-location where different programmes are placed in the same setting.

Information and referral systems.

Central intake and referral providing a single point of access.

Inter-agency networks that create specific linkages between programmes. Three types are described:
    a. Multidisciplinary teams
    b. Bilateral coordination
    c. Multilateral coordination

Case management.

Sharing of staff.

Financing models.

Education and training.

There needs to be a range of drug-related services offered in the community. My colleague designed a graphic representation of how a continuum of care and the process and components of treatment might look for drug users with multiple problems (see Figure 1 and Figure 2).

In considering what skills and competencies were required, we developed a list of services that we felt needed to be available for all those who have concerns related to drug use:

RANGE OF SERVICES REQUIRED

Drop-in services such as day care.

Brief, time-limited interventions.

Low threshold, harm reduction services providing information, advice, and support in reducing drug-related concerns and harm (e.g. needle exchanges, injection site assessment, HIV and hepatitis and safer sex services). Assessment of drug-related concerns and issues. Joint assessment tools enhance the ability of programmes to coordinate services. Standardised assessment instruments are recommended with additional instruments to provide information unique to individual programmes. Assessment should include all drug use patterns as well as biological, psychological, and social issues.

Education on available treatment options (including strengths and limitations).

Drug counselling guided by individualised needs assessment, and treatment planning.

Maintenance of change and relapse prevention work.

Case management of social issues (e.g. budgeting, housing, child care, etc.).

Issues affecting mental health (anxiety; depression; hopelessness; past/present physical or sexual abuse; stress management and coping strategies; parental drug issues; sleep, anger, and grief issues; problem solving; psychiatric issues, etc.).

Medical assessment and management (including pain, hepatitis, and HIV issues).

Prescribing issues. Substitute prescribing may be appropriate in some cases.

Prescribing services may also be a part of a detox programme or for psychiatric issues.

Dietary and nutrition issues.

Social support systems and relationship issues (couples, families, friends).

Family history (social, drug use, criminality and mental health).

Parenting and child-care issues (including pregnancy).

Crisis intervention services.

Sexuality issues.

Gender specific issues.

Legal issues.

Educational and vocational issues.

Recreational issues.

Daily living issues (e.g. personal hygiene, household tasks, cooking, shopping, etc).

Social skills training (e.g. assertiveness and communication skills, etc.).

Given the diversity of needs, we can see why close collaboration is required across many disciplines. The following is not an exhaustive list but includes the major areas:

DISCIPLINES INVOLVED WITH DRUG WORK

Counselling • Social Work • Nursing (psychiatric and general)

Psychiatry • Psychology • Religious and Spiritual Guides

General Practice • Family Therapists

Physiotherapy • Occupational Health •

Acupuncture and Alternative Interventions

Education (School and Community) • Child Care Staff

Pharmacists • Police and Prison Officers

As stated earlier, the inclusion of the entire community, from drug users and their families to community and self-help groups, will be fundamental in moving 'beyond maintenance'. Again, the importance of close collaboration with these groups cannot be underestimated.

Figure 1   A PICTURE OF DRUG SERVICES IN THE COMMUNITY
Serving the Drug, Mental Health and Social Needs of People with Drug Problems

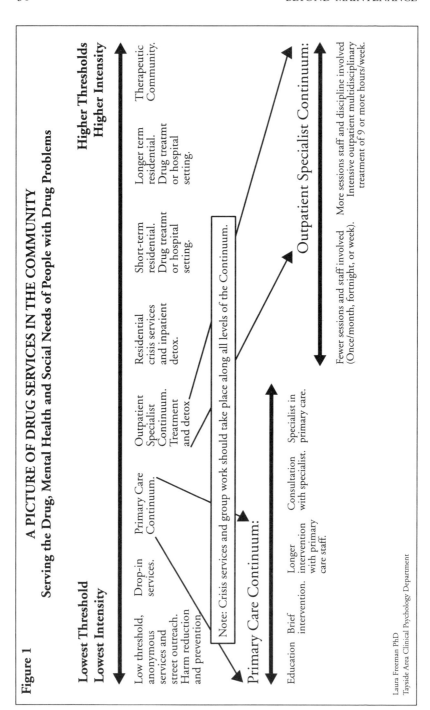

Laura Freeman PhD
Tayside Area Clinical Psychology Department

Figure 2

HELPING CLIENTS WITH MULTIPLE ISSUES: AN INTEGRATED FRAMEWORK FOR DRUG AND ALCOHOL TREATMENT

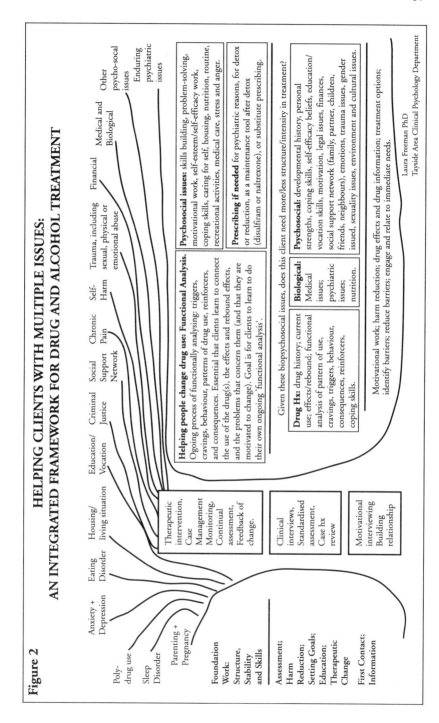

Laura Freeman PhD
Tayside Area Clinical Psychology Department

References

Abram, K. M., and L. A. Teplin. 1991. Co-occurring disorders among mentally ill jail detainees: Implication for public policy. *American Psychologist* 46, 1036-1045.

Appleby, L., V. Dyson, E. Altman, and D. Luchins. 1997. Assessing substance use in multi problem patients: Reliability and validity of the Addiction Severity Index in a mental hospital population. *Journal of Nervous and Mental Disease* 185, 159-165.

Bannister, A., 1992. Working with adult female survivors of childhood sexual abuse. In *Hearing to Healing*. NSPPC: Longman.

Barbee, J. G., P. D. Clark, M. S. Crapanzano, G. C. Heintz, and C. E. Kehoe. 1989. Alcohol and substance abuse among schizophrenic patients presenting to emergency psychiatric services. *Journal of Nervous and Mental Disease* 177, 400-407.

Bartles, S. J., R. E. Drake, M. A. Wallach, and D. H. Freeman. 1991. Characteristic hostility in schizophrenic outpatients. *Schizophrenia Bulletin,* 163-171.

Bernstein, David P., Judith A. Stein, and Leonard Handelman. 1998. Predicting personality pathology among adult patients with substance use disorders: effects of childhood maltreatment. *Addictive Behaviours,* 855-868.

Brady, K., T. Killeen, M. Saladin, B. Dansky, and S. Becker. 1994. Comorbid substance abuse and post-traumatic stress disorder: Characteristics of women in treatment. *The American Journal on Addictions* 3(2), 160-164.

Briere, J. 1992. *Child Abuse Trauma: Theory and Treatment of the Lasting Effects.* Newbury Park, CA: Sage.

Brown, P., R. Stout, and T. Mueller. 1996. Post-traumatic stress disorder and substance abuse relapse among women: A pilot study. *Psychology of Addictive Behaviours* 10, 124.

Brown, P. J., and J. Wolfe. 1994. Substance abuse and post-traumatic stress disorder comorbidity. *Drug and Alcohol Dependence* 35, 51-59.

Chiles, J. A., E. Von Cleve, R. P. Jemelka, and E. W. Trupin. 1990. Substance abuse and psychiatric disorders in prison inmates. *Hospital and Community Psychiatry* 41, 1132-1134.

Copeland, J., and W. Hall. 1992. A comparison of women seeking drug and alcohol treatment in a specialist women's and two traditional mixed-sex treatment services. *British Journal of Addiction* 87, 67-74.

Coryell, W., J. Endicott, and G. Winokur. 1992. Anxiety syndromes as epiphenomena of primary depression: Outcome and familial psychopathology. *American Journal of Psychiatry* 149, 100-107.

Dansky B., M. Saladin, K. Brady, D. Kilpatrick and H. Resnick 1995. Post-traumatic stress disorders among substance users from the general population *The International Journal of the Addictions* 30, 1079-1099.

Derks, J. 1990. The Amsterdam Morphine Dispensing Programme. A longitudinal study of extremely problematic drug addicts in an experimental public health programme. *NcGv-series, no 90-3,* Utrecht, the Netherlands.

Drake, R. E., and M. F. Brunette. 1998. Complications of severe mental illness relation to alcohol and drug use disorders. In *Recent Developments in Alcoholism,* ed. M. Galanter, Vol 14: 285-299. New York: Plenum.

Fullilove M., R. Fillilove, M. Smith, K. Winkler, C. Michael, P. Panzer, and R. Wallace. 1993. Violence, trauma and post-traumatic stress disorder among women drug users. *Journal of Traumatic Stress* 6(4), 533-543.

Gil-Rivas V., R. Fiorentine, and M. D. Anglin. 1996. Sexual abuse, physical abuse and post-traumatic stress disorder among women participating in outpatient drug abuse treatment. *Journal of Psychoactive Drugs* 28(1), 95-102.

Hendricks, V. M. 1990. Psychiatric disorders in a Dutch addict population: Rates and correlates of SAM-III diagnoses. *Journal of Consulting and Clinical Psychology* 58, 158-165.

Jarvis T., and J. Copeland. 1997. Child sexual abuse as a predictor of psychiatric co-morbidity and its implications for drug and alcohol treatment. *Drug and Alcohol Dependence* 49, 61-69.

Jemelka, R., E. Trupin, and J. Chiles. 1989. The mentally ill in prisons: A review. *Hospital and Community Psychiatry* 40, 481-491 (1993).

Johnson, S. 1997. Dual diagnosis of severe mental illness and substance misuse: A case for specialist services? *British Journal of Psychiatry* 171, 205-208.

Kessler, R. C., R. M. Crum, L. A. Warner, C. B. Nelson, J. Schulenberg, and J. C. Anthony. 1997. Lifetime co-occurrence of DSM-III-R alcohol abuse and dependence with other psychiatric disorders in the National Comorbidity Survey. *Archives of General Psychiatry* 54, 313-321.

Kokkevi A., N. Stefanis, E. Anastasopoulou, and C. Kostogianni. 1998.

Personality Disorders in drug abusers: prevalence and their association with Axis I Disorders as predictors of treatment retention. *Addictive Behaviours* 23, 841-853.

Krausz, M., P. K. Degkwitz, A. Kuhne, and U. Verthein. 1998. Co-morbidity of opiate dependence and mental disorders. *Addictive Behaviours* 23, 767-783.

Kulka, R. A., W. E. Schlenger, J. A. Fairbank, R. L. Hough, B. K. Jordan, C. R. Marmar, and D. S. Weiss. 1990. *Trauma and the Vietnam War Generation: Report of Findings from the National Vietnam Veterans Readjustment Study.* New York: Brunner/Mazel.

Lucks, N. 1997. HMP Cornton Vale: Research into drugs and alcohol violence, bullying, suicides, self-injury and backgrounds of abuse. Scottish Prison Service Occasional Papers: Report No. 1/98. HMSO: London Cornton Vale.

Miller, B., W. Downs, D. Gondoli, and A. Keil. (1987). The role of childhood sexual abuse in the development of alcoholism in women. *Violence and Victims* 3, 157-172.

Miller B., W. Downs, and M. Testa. 1993. Interrelationships between victimisation experiences and women's alcohol use. *Journal of Studies on Alcohol* 11(11), 109-117.

Mueser, K. T., A. S. Bellack, and J. J. Blanchard. 1992. Co-morbidity of schizophrenia and substance abuse: Implications for treatment. *Journal of Consulting and Clinical Psychology* 60(6), 845-856.

Najavits, Lisa M., Roger D. Weis, Sarah R. Shaw, and Larry R. Muenz. 1998. 'Seeking Safety': Outcome of a new cognitive-behavioural psychotherapy for women with post-traumatic stress disorder and substance dependence. *Journal of Traumatic Stress* 11(3), 437-456.

Osher, F. C., and L. L. Kofoed. 1989. Treatment of patients with psychiatric and psychoactive substance abuse disorders. *Hospital and Community Psychiatry* 40, 1025-1030.

Paone, D., W. Chavking, I. Willets, P. Friedman, and D. DesJarlais. 1992. The impact of sexual abuse: implications for treatment. *Journal of Women's Health* 1, 149-153.

Porter, S. 1993. Assault experiences among drug users. *Substance Abuse Bulletin* 8.

Ravdnal, E., and P. Vaglum. 1995. The influence of personality disorders on treatment completion in a hierarchical therapeutic community for drug abusers: A prospective study. *European Addiction Research* 1, 178-186.

Regier, D., M. Farmer, D. Rae, B. Locke, S. Keith, L. Judd, and F. Goodwin. (1990). Comorbidity of mental disorders with alcohol and other drug abuse: Results from the Epidemiologic Catchment Area (ECA) Study. *Journal of the American Medical Association* 264, 2511-2518.

Rohsenow, D. J., R. Corbett, and D. Devine. 1988. Molested as children: A hidden contribution to substance abuse? *Journal of Substance Abuse* 5.

Sacks, S., and G. De Leon. 1997. *Modified therapeutic community for homeless mentally ill chemical abusers: profiles, process and outcomes.* Paper presented at the American Psychological Association annual meeting, Chicago.

Safer, D. J. 1987. Substance abuse by chronic adult patients. *Hospital and Community Psychiatry* 38, 511-514.

Scott, J., E. Gilvarry, and M. Farrell. 1998. Managing anxiety and depression in alcohol and drug dependence. *Addictive Behaviours* 23, 919-913.

Simpson, Tracy L., Verner S. Westerberg, Laura M. Little, and Margie Trujillo. 1994. Screening for childhood physical and sexual abuse among outpatient substance abusers. *Journal of Substance Abuse Treatment* 11(4), 347-358.

Stewart, S. H. 1996. Alcohol abuse in individuals exposed to trauma: A critical review. *Psychological Bulletin* 120(1), 83-112.

Trotter, C. 1992. Stages of recovery and relapse prevention for the chemically dependent adult sexual trauma survivor. In *Treatment Innovations,* ed., M. Hunter. London: Sage.

Wallace, C., P. Mullen, P. Burgess, S. Palmer, D. Ruschena, and C. Browne. 1998. Serious criminal offending and mental disorders. *British Journal of Psychiatry* 172, 477-484.

Wilson, J. A. 1997. Childhood Sexual Abuse and Adult Dependence: The Connection. *Druglink* 12(3). Institute for the Study of Drug Dependence, London.

Yandow, V. 1989. Alcoholism in Women. *Psychiatric Annals 19.*

Zeirler, S., L. Feingold, D. Laufer, P. Velentgas, G. Kantrowitz, and K. Mayer. 1991. Adult survivors of childhood sexual abuse and subsequent risk of HIV infection. *American Journal of Public Health* 81.

Minister Eoin Ryan

As Minister with special responsibility for the National Drugs Strategy, I am delighted to have this opportunity to address this seminar. With an overall review of the National Drugs Strategy currently under way, today's seminar comes at a very opportune time in the development of policy in relation to drug treatment.

The principal aim of this review is to ensure that the policies and strategies that we are currently pursuing remain relevant to the situation as it exists on the ground. The review will examine the extent and nature of the drug problem nationally, identify any major gaps and deficiencies in the current response to the problem, and make recommendations on how the strategy can be modified to address these gaps and deficiencies.

As part of the review, my Department has undertaken a series of consultative fora at a number of different locations around the country. The fora provided a valuable opportunity for all those working in the drugs field to have an input into how our policy should be shaped for the future. We have also invited submissions from interested individuals and groups, and, to date, we have received over 160.

The deliberations of this seminar will hopefully serve to further inform the review process and I would invite you to make a submission to the review in the light of your discussions today.

Judging from the packed itinerary set out for the day, the conference will provide ample opportunity to examine the range of issues associated with the provision of effective drug treatment services for drug users. The guest speakers this morning, coming as they do from various backgrounds and disciplines, provided some invaluable insights on issues around drug misuse and I'm sure they gave you much food for thought.

The Government is determined to tackle the drug problem in

Ireland and we have committed very significant resources to achieve this. Over £1 billion is earmarked to implement social inclusion measures in the new National Development Plan, including initiatives to respond to the drug problem.

A comprehensive package of measures have been put in place to tackle the problem. We have brought forward legislation to increase the powers of the Gardaí and other authorities to tackle organised crime and drug dealing. The Criminal Assets Bureau, in particular, is seen as an extremely effective weapon in our armoury against the drug barons. We are now denying these thugs the opportunity to enjoy the wealth they have amassed through inflicting misery on the lives of others.

However, as those working with drug users know only too well, we cannot solve the problem simply by cutting off the supply of drugs. We must also put in place measures to prevent young people from turning to drugs in the first instance, as well as treatment and rehabilitation options for those who are already addicted. We have made very significant strides in this regard over the past few years. The numbers in treatment, for example, have risen from around 1,400 in 1996 to nearly 5,000 this year. While we have not yet reached the stage where we have eliminated waiting lists, I am confident we are moving in that direction. More and more drug users are presenting for treatment as services expand and improve, and that, in itself, is a positive development. The more people we can encourage into treatment the better.

Some people argue that there may be as many as 13,000 heroin users in Dublin and that only about a third of them are in treatment. The reality, however, is that not all heroin users are ready to present at any given time. Our aim must be to make sure that when they do, the services are there. The Eastern Regional Health Authority (ERHA) – in whose area the vast majority of heroin users reside – estimate that if they provide a further five or six treatment centres, they will be very close to eliminating waiting lists. Their drug service plan for 2000 is geared towards this aim.

Of course, we should not wait for drug users to present. We must actively encourage them to do so, in their own interest and in the interests of society generally. To address this, we have appointed outreach workers to attract addicts into treatment. Through the Local Drugs Task Forces, we have set up support and advice centres for drug users and their families. Indeed, over 4,000 users and 3,000 families have availed of these services to date.

It is worth noting that the ERHA and the Prison Service have also developed a joint programme of action aimed at ensuring that the level of treatment available to drug users inside prison is consistent with that available on the outside. Obviously, when drug users are committed to prison, it presents an ideal opportunity to get them thinking in terms of doing something about their addiction. It is important that the facilities and services are in place to respond to this opportunity.

In addition, proposals have been developed for a pilot drug court system, which will offer treatment and rehabilitation options to drug users as an alternative to a prison sentence. Again, this is a time when drug users are most likely to be thinking about changing their lifestyle.

There has been much debate about the use of methadone in the treatment of drug use. My own view is that a range of options and treatment interventions are necessary. Methadone is a very effective intervention, as evidenced by the fact that nearly 300,000 drug users around Europe are on this form of treatment. However, I feel strongly that it must be backed up by a range of other services, such as counselling and training, if it is to be effective in the long term. Our aim is to provide these support services with a view to moving as many people as possible towards being drug free.

A very encouraging trend is the number of people on methadone who are finding employment. A recent study of the Health Board's treatment services found that almost 40 per cent of those on methadone were now working. This proves that, with treatment and other supports, drug users can return to a full and normal life. Nearly 700 drug users are now in specially designed Community Employment schemes, which offer them counselling, training and other necessary supports.

The Task Forces have been allocated £15 million, on top of an earlier £10 million, to update their drug action plans. They are being asked to develop more rehabilitation programmes in the new plans. While I will not be satisfied until every drug user in the country has ready access to treatment and rehabilitation, I think it is fair to say that, by international comparisons, we have made astounding progress in developing our services over the past few years.

This has been done in some instances against a background of opposition to the setting up of satellite clinics, often as a result of fear or misapprehension on the part of local residents. As a society, we owe every citizen the right to a full and happy life. We owe it to drug users to try to understand more about the nature of their addiction and to offer whatever supports we can to help them to overcome it.

The importance of education in combating drug misuse has been highlighted at each of the consultative fora I spoke about earlier. Through the Task Forces, nearly 350 schools have had drug awareness programmes, with nearly 6,000 school children participating in these programmes. 350 teachers have received training, over 300 youth groups have run drug prevention initiatives, while training programmes have been delivered to 1,300 community workers, 1,200 parents, and 1,300 young people outside the school setting.

Sport and leisure can play a vital role in diverting young people away from drugs and into healthier pursuits. Through the Young People's Facilities and Services Fund, we are supporting the building or refurbishment of nearly 50 youth facilities, 20 sports clubs and nearly 20 community centres. Almost 80 youth and outreach workers are being appointed to work with young people at risk of becoming involved in drugs.

These are just some of the interventions that are currently being put in place. However, I think it is important to acknowledge that it will take time for many of these measures to impact fully. The drug problem will not be solved overnight. Drug misuse is a complex problem requiring a multi-disciplinary response across a range of agencies and professions. Collectively we must build on the good work that has been done to date and increase our resolve and commitment to control this great social ill that affects many of our communities.

I would like to take this opportunity today to express my sincere appreciation for the commitment, energy and expertise that members of the clergy have brought to bear in addressing the drug problem, and social inclusion issues generally, both nationally and at a local level. The range and depth of their involvement is tremendous, from prevention and education, through all areas of treatment and rehabilitation, to policy development at a national level. The Church has often shown great leadership in this area and I hope it will continue to play an important role in gaining acceptance for treatment clinics and other supports in local communities.

The support and participation of the Church in the development and delivery of the current response to the drug problem has been a key factor in the significant progress achieved to date. Today's seminar is yet further evidence of the priority that the Church attaches to the development of an effective response to the drugs issue and to promoting informed debate on overall policy.

Recognising the importance of sound research and analysis as a guide to both policy formulation and the design and delivery of effective services, I am very pleased to announce that the Government is establishing a National Advisory Committee on Drugs.

This new Committee will advise the Government in relation to the prevalence, prevention, treatment and consequences of problem drug use in Ireland, based on its analysis and interpretation of research findings and information available to it. The Committee will also oversee the delivery of a three-year research programme aimed at addressing priority information gaps and deficiencies, including issues relating to the effectiveness of existing treatment and rehabilitation models and programmes. This Committee will, I'm sure, prove to be an invaluable resource for policy-makers, service providers and the general public alike.

I intend to establish the Committee in July.

RESPONSE TO JANE WILSON PAPER

Dr Desmond Corrigan

The most welcome paper by Jane Wilson highlights yet again the complex, multifaceted nature of what is commonly called 'the drug problem'. This term has always seemed a misnomer because it implies that all drugs are similar, that all drug users are similar, and that all drug use takes place within similar family, community or cultural settings. Dr Wilson has shown us clearly that not only are all those who use drugs different, they also present with a bewildering array of problems among which she highlights those of post-traumatic stress disorder and dual diagnosis. She highlights the need for a complex, multifaceted, multi-disciplinary response to the myriad of difficulties presented by such individuals.

In a presentation full of information and provocative challenges and ideas, certain key themes stand out and I have chosen to concentrate on these. They are:

1. Territorial boundaries
2. What works with what clients
3. Dual diagnosis
4. Self-medication
5. The holistic approach

Territorial Boundaries
This phrase was used in the context of multi-disciplinary teamwork among the caring agencies and professions. In this country these boundaries are being progressively eroded and blurred through the Integrated Services Project and through the Local Drugs Task Forces, where the demarcation between community and statutory is slowly but surely disappearing and where the statutory agencies themselves are learning the value of interagency cooperation. The linkage of community and statutory through the Drug Task Forces locally and

through the National Drug Strategy Team nationally, is a unique feature of the Irish system and it harnesses strengths and resources we often underestimate or even don't realise we have. Often we believe that we are behind everyone else, when the reality is that we are ahead of our EU neighbours in some areas and no different in others.

That is not to say that we cannot learn from the experiences of others, we can and must.

What works with what clients
This is one of those areas where we can learn from other countries. We do need to recognise that a variety of treatment options are necessary. Personally I have always had great difficulty with the concept of treatment 'slots', which conveys to me the idea of slotting individuals into a conveyor-belt treatment process, when the treatment programme should ideally be built round the individual. The art should be to find which treatment is most appropriate for a given individual at a given point in their drug-using career.

We need to have available a range of both pharmacological *and* non-pharmacological interventions. I emphasise the 'and' in that last sentence because both are needed. It is quite clear from evaluations of treatment outcomes in other countries that no one treatment 'modality', to use the jargon, is superior or pre-eminent. We should not be afraid to use the range of pharmacological treatments available for detoxification, maintenance and relapse prevention. Some would oppose this approach because of its reliance on chemicals in a situation of chemical dependency, but many drug users are either not ready or not able to maintain abstinence, and in such cases medication has a role to play.

The impact of the 'self-medication' theory needs to be taken on board in this context. We also urgently need to discover if it is the 'self-medicators', out of increasingly large numbers of hedonistic drug users, who are at highest risk of developing dependence and the whole range of other drug-related problems. Not only do we need to use existing medications such as methadone and lofexidine, but we also need to investigate the usefulness of LAAM, buprenorphine and naltrexone among others. Even more importantly, we must encourage efforts to develop new treatments for addictions based on our new knowledge of the molecular biology of the human brain (Litten and

Allen 1999). We must see methadone for what it is – a part of the process, or, to paraphrase Winston Churchill, 'it is perhaps the beginning of the beginning' of the road to recovery.

Combined with the use of supportive medicines, we must have a variety of non-pharmacological treatments such as psychotherapy, including cognitive-behavioural therapy and psychodynamic approaches, therapeutic communities, 12-step recovery programmes, and even good old-fashioned religion! We need to encourage and foster innovation and alternatives, but in a manner that allows each therapy to be properly evaluated. This of course presupposes an evaluation mechanism and this surely will be a key task of the new National Advisory Committee, to be established by the government. We do urgently need a mechanism similar to the National Treatment Outcome Research Survey (NTORS) in the UK.

We need to understand too that we are dealing with a range of addictive substances and not just opiates, that our treatment programmes need to be able to respond to the needs of those addicted to benzodiozepines, stimulants, cannabis and also to those with 'multiple dependencies', for example, to opiates and alcohol.

Dual diagnosis

If individuals with multiple dependencies present a challenge to services, then those with the dual diagnosis of addiction and co-existing psychiatric disorders present an even more formidable challenge.

The reason for this lies in the fact that the same chemical pathways in the brain that have been linked to the addictive use of drugs including alcohol have also been implicated in the development of mental disorders such as schizophrenia and bipolar disorders. It is increasingly recognised that using medication for these disorders may have an affect on the addictive disorders (Pechter and Miller 1997, 23-40).

Experts on dual diagnosis emphasise the need for proper diagnosis, since drug use may obscure the diagnosis. They recommend that abstinence should first be achieved before it is possible to state that the symptoms are due to a non-drug psychiatric disorder and not just due to the drug use itself. This abstinence, of course, is well recognised as being difficult to achieve and maintain, and thus a 'catch 22' situation may be created. In addition, those working with drug users with a potential dual diagnosis need to be aware that certain drugs will not only obscure the diagnosis, but may in fact exacerbate the symptoms. I have in mind the paranoid symptoms associated with cocaine and amphetamine, the depressive effects of alcohol, the psychotic symptoms linked to LSD and the way in which cannabis use precipitates and exacerbates existing schizophrenic states.

On the other hand it must be emphasised that methadone maintenance is not contra-indicated and in fact the evidence suggests that some depressive disorders remit. Others do not and require psychotherapy or anti-depressant medication or both. It is important that patients are not deprived of appropriate medication but at the same time inappropriate medication, for example, benzodiazepines, can be devastating in its effects. In this connection the proposal to develop a protocol for benzodiazepine prescribing deserves a hearty welcome. With regard to heroin, it is noteworthy that the external evaluation of the Swiss heroin-prescribing study reported that it was of limited value in multiple dependence or in the dually diagnosed (WHO 1999).

Extent of Dual Diagnosis in Ireland
The standard sources of information on problem drug use, for example, the Statistical Bulletin of the National Drug Treatment Reporting System (NDTRS) published by the Health Research Board, do not contain information on the extent of this aspect of the problem. The external evaluation of the Drugs/AIDS Services of the old Eastern Health Board does mention the fact that 14 per cent of urines from clients in different treatment clinics tested positive for tricyclics, which are just one class of anti-depressant. This gives a partial clue to the existence of the phenomenon but since the figures do not include any of the newer SSRI type anti-depressants, they are incomplete (Eastern Health Board 2000). Many people have drawn attention to the high level of urines positive for benzodiazepines. One could be charitable and interpret this as evidence of significant levels of anxiety states in such patients, but inappropriate prescribing and outright abuse seem more obvious explanations. It is clear therefore that we do need some research into the extent of psychiatric co-

morbidity/dual diagnosis in Ireland. It is to be hoped that the National Advisory Committee, through its research remit, might examine this. Internationally, much of the work has been of US origin. The Annual Report on the State of the Drugs Problem in the EU, published by the European Monitoring Centre for Drugs and Drug Addiction (EMCDDA), to be published later this year, will report that only the Netherlands and Sweden report dual diagnosis as a significant issue. What we have learnt at this seminar suggests that it needs a greater priority attached to it at European level in the context of the new three-year work programme to be adopted later this year.

The External Review of the Eastern Health Board (EHB) did draw attention to the possible impact of dual diagnosis (page 30) when it noted 'the presence of psychiatric co-morbidity amongst drug users has been linked to poorer outcomes'. However the report did indicate a possible response in Recommendation 7.18:

> Given the integrated nature of EHB services there seems to be a strong case for substantial expansion in this form of liaison/shared care model into primary care, general mental health services, child and adolescent psychiatric services, hepatology services and criminal justice agencies. At a local level, case managers or liaison workers could provide a key role in ensuring that a combination of community and statutory resources are mobilised in order to achieve maximum treatment and rehabilitation impact. (Eastern Health Board 2000)

Holistic Approaches

This recommendation, if it was implemented through either the key worker, case manager, or liaison worker routes would certainly go a long way to ensuring that the multiple needs of problem drug users can be met. It is questionable however if drugs workers have the skills, or indeed should be expected to have the skills, to assess dual diagnosis, or if they are in a position to provide a sort of 'one-stop response shop' for the multitude of medical, psychiatric, legal, social and educational difficulties encountered by drug users. For example, the Dun Laoghaire-Rathdown Local Drugs Task Force recently commissioned a survey of clients in rehabilitation in order to establish their needs in the context of a revised action plan. A major but less than surprising finding was that literacy levels were at a very low level in the population surveyed. Rehabilitation of such clients must overcome this major hurdle if these individuals are to be fully reintegrated into society. It will be essential that individual workers have a broad base of skills and access to a broad range of services for their clients.

Service developments that are coming on stream and those that are planned, do offer the prospect of seamless care for problem drug users. There is an increasing awareness, reinforced by Dr Wilson's presentation, that addicts do not constitute a homogenous population and that treatment plans must be individualised.

Her exposition of the complexity of the problems faced by drug users, their families and communities, highlights the need to educate policy-makers of the necessity for a long-term commitment, because there are no easy, cheap or quick solutions to a problem that is chronic and relapsing.

The existing non-party political consensus must be maintained and nourished, especially when the financial outlook becomes less positive at some stage in the future. Presentations such as those by Dr Wilson are of enormous value in maintaining awareness of the complexity of the drugs issue and of the futility of simplistic responses.

References

External Review of Drug Services for the Eastern Health Board. January 2000. Farrell, M., C. Gerada, and J. Marsden.

Litten, R. and J. P. J. Allen. 1999. Medications for Alcohol, Illicit Drug and Tobacco Dependence: An update of research findings. *Substance Abuse Treatment* 16 (2) 105-112.

Pechter, B. N., and S. Miller. 1997. Psychopharmacology for Addictive and Comorbid Disorders: Current Studies. In *The Integration of Pharmacological and Nonpharmacological Treatments in Drug/Alcohol Addictions,* ed., Miller, N. New York: Haworth Medical Press.

WHO. April 1999. Report of the external panel on the evaluation of the Swiss Scientific Studies of Medically prescribed Narcotics to Drug Addicts.

QUESTIONS AND ANSWERS

Panel: Dr Des Corrigan, Jane Wilson, Anna Quigley, Minister Eoin Ryan
Chairperson: Chris Murphy

Topic: Child-Care Facilities

Q. [Questioner unidentified]: The treatment I'm in now is day treatment and even at that there's nowhere for my baby. I have to make my own arrangements.

A: Ms Jane Wilson: In Scotland there are two rehabilitation units that take in parents and children for a period of six months. Specialist workers are brought in to work with children in the day while drug workers work with the mothers. I know there are some in England as well, but certainly those two are the only two available in Scotland. It is an issue, because if a woman was to go into rehab and has children there's a fear of abandoning the children when going for services – those children need support as well.

A: Ms Anna Quigley: About £250 million has now been allocated to child care under a new scheme by the Department of Justice. One of the important things we have to do is to meet with the Department of Justice and make sure that a certain amount of that child-care money is allocated to the people who are running the drug services, because in all drug services, particularly the community-based services, the lack of any kind of child-care facility is a huge issue. They've been trying to get child-care facilities but the Task Force and the Health Board have always felt, 'Well, that's not our brief'.

A: Minister Eoin Ryan: Just to support what Anna said, £250 million has been allocated for crèche facilities in areas that suffer from social exclusion. It is for those areas. I think we have to make sure it is targeted in the right way. You can throw money at problems and if it is not put in place properly then it can be wasted and we'd find out in a few years' time that we're not getting the services that we need in the proper places.

Comment: Mr Denis Murray: I think that children going to school should be supported. If there were supports available for them at times of crisis in their life, then we could give them the care that they need. There have been a huge numbers of deaths – communities are suffering the haemorrhage of death and deprivation and are unable to lift themselves out of it – and methadone is not the solution because it suppresses a rage at what's happening around them, which should have an outlet.

Topic: Treatment or Prison?
Q: Mr Steve Jones: Why is it that the main focus of treatment by this government and by succeeding governments (and by the society we live in) is detention? Maybe we could have some feedback on it from the panel.

A: Minister Eoin Ryan: Well, I don't think the main focus of treatment is detention. We've set up the drug courts so that people will have an alternative. What we're trying to do is put proper prisons in place with proper services in those prisons where you can treat prisoners properly. But also, there was a revolving-door syndrome, which there was public outrage about. People wanted us to respond to it and we did. Certainly that gives us an opportunity to treat and to deal with prisoners far more humanely and far more intelligently than has been the case up to now. Either we can fill those prisons with more and more people, which I don't think we will, or we can use the situation, first of all, to get drugs out of the prison, and also to give more rehabilitation and education facilities in there. That's certainly what I'd be looking for.

Topic: Financial Provision for Services
Q: Mr David Clinch: Is it the case that our society is not able to provide some shelter or place for people who are of the gentler persuasion anymore? Is there a case not just for treatment and

secondary treatment, but for tilting the Celtic Tiger say 10 per cent on its axis to somewhere that the market doesn't go, where labels of success are not always in the financial area?

A: Ms Anna Quigley: I think it's something that we keep saying in terms of this Celtic Tiger, because in some ways the fact that there is prosperity in parts of the country has given the message that in some way or other, prosperity is the answer to all our problems. It's clear to us that there are certain services and certain supports that we have to provide to people as a society. It's a mark of what we are as a society. It's not about whether we can afford them or whether we can't afford them. We have a responsibility as a society to spend our money – taxpayers' money – in a way that supports people who need our support, whenever they need it, whether they be drug users, people with illnesses, or with psychiatric problems.

Q: Ms Marie Dillon: When we start to peel the onion of addiction, what we find is homelessness, child care difficulties, and the fact that in the Tower rehab project where I work, the only vehicle we have to operate on is a FAS community employment scheme. Now while we are grateful for that, it is very confusing for people who come to recovery on a FAS community employment scheme. They perceive this to be work, and they perceive the payment to be a reward for work done in a twenty-hour-per-week period. Also, men who come to these programmes are discriminated against in that they do not have lone parent books and they received only their CE funding. I'm wondering if the Minister could possibly look at ways of assisting these people to avail of recovery and rehabilitation aside from community employment?

Q: Ms Trish Williams: I'd ask the Minister to put more money into family support, as it does great work. The housing problem also makes it hard for people who come out of treatment.

Q: Ms Áine Walsh: A dirty school, a dirty home, a waiting list for treatment, says to a person: you do not matter as much as somebody in a different part of town that has more advantage. So as a society we need to look at the global aspect of it. It's a massive social ill, not just a 'drug problem'. The minister should contact all the other ministers, looking for educational change, social welfare change, housing change, medical change.

A: Ms Jane Wilson: Social cohesion means recognising that those of us who do well need to care for all our children in society. We all have this responsibility and if we begin to fragment into those who do well and continue to marginalise those who don't, the gaps and the problems will increase right across the sectors. Your prisons will be overflowing and your mental hospitals will be overflowing. Social cohesion does require a bridging and a recognition that there does have to be a level playing-field for all our people.

A: Minister Eoin Ryan: The Cabinet sub-committee on social inclusion meets every month; I go, and so does the Department of Health, Education, Environment, Social Welfare, Justice, and Finance, and the Taoiseach himself chairs it. It deals exclusively with issues of social exclusion – exactly what you're talking about. I'll give you an example: Two principals of schools came to me and said 'We've one problem: I'm losing one teacher and this principal is losing another.' Tomorrow at the social exclusion committee meeting I have this on the agenda. So there is a mechanism there to tackle this.

A: Ms Anna Quigley: Just to respond to a couple of the points that came up. On family support, I very strongly agree that one of the very positive things that has happened in the absence of services for families is that families themselves have come together and are offering each other support. But again that is going to need resourcing. Just because it's families doesn't mean it can be done on fresh air.

About the Community Employment schemes, FÁS obviously are part of the national strategy and they've been asked to play a role in it, and they have CE funding. We need to look at it in a broader way and say, well we have the basic model of CE and now that needs to be adapted and developed in a way that actually suits the needs of drug users. You can't just use it off the shelf.

Topic: Involvement of Drug Users in Policy Decisions

Q: Mr Richie Bracken: You would never have a recovering addict or a well addict on these committees or advisory boards, you know, someone who has in-depth experience. Who better to know?

A: Ms Anna Quigley: In response to Richie's question, it has come up at the review of the NDST [National Drug Strategy Team] that up to now the target group of the NDST hasn't been involved, and that's been highlighted.

A: Minister Eoin Ryan: I have met a lot of recovering addicts throughout the country and in residential, I do want to meet a lot of addicts as part of the review, just to talk to them about how they see the problem they're dealing with every single day.

A: Dr. Des Corrigan: To Richie, in our own drug task force a study was conducted which was very much the voice of addicts in recovery and what they want and what they need; and that will more than inform – it will decide our strategy in terms of rehabilitation. I know that it's part of the existing rehab project, that the users know the pain and have an impact on the management and decision-making process, as it should be. I think that in many of the task forces, this is going on in a low-key way.

Topic: Pharmacology and Alternative Therapies

Q: Mr Val Keaveney: I'm a community representative on the Dun Laoghaire Local Drugs Task Force and my question is to Dr Des Corrigan. Now I know you do not have a crystal ball, but recognising yesterday's announcement in the field of DNA genetic mapping, would you foresee that, at some future time, some pharmaceutical company could develop a drug that would give almost instant detoxification and remove the residual longing and cravings of the addicted person?

A: Dr. Des Corrigan: I don't know that I would go that far, but I do think there will be quite new treatments for all kinds of addictions that will come out of the kinds of molecular biology research we're seeing.

I don't think we'll get the big 'wham' type result that you envisage but it will make a difference in the lives of people who are affected by addictions, which might be one of the advantages of research that third-level work might bring about.

Q: Ms Martina Dow: I just wonder if it ever strikes you that the reason why people become addicted or become mentally unwell in terms of schizophrenia or manic depression is because they're suffering from a severe lack of love and emotional support in their lives; and the way forward is not by giving them drugs but good old-fashioned love? Your industry is such that there is an 80 per cent mark-up on your drugs. And psychiatrists working with you seem to become drug dispensers. Basically what I'm saying is that the business you're running is an inhuman and criminal one and I think you should look at what you are doing very carefully.

A: Dr. Des Corrigan: I am not a spokesperson for the pharmaceutical industry. Can I just say that many in this room, myself included, would not be alive today if it weren't for the advances in modern medicine and in modern pharmacy. It is easy to criticise things that go wrong. The difficulty that you deal with when dealing with drugs is that they are inherently dangerous chemicals and there will always be side effects and there will always be problems.

A: Ms Jane Wilson: In the history of psychiatry and the use of pharmacology it is well known that up to now some have been particularly beneficial. There needs to be some balance there. Some of the newer drugs – Prozac (when it is not excessively used) or sleeping medication, or non-addictive medication – can provide support to someone who is addicted, struggling through recovery and not able to sleep. However, there is a history of over-medication where it's used as a control mechanism rather than more intensive therapeutic interventions and so we do need to watch that space carefully.

Q: Fr Joe Pereira: I asked the Lord to guide me and in the morning he told me to shut up, but this afternoon, if I may say something about our work in India, it's the meditation along with a little medication. Just as the drug is capable of making a pathway into the brain, we in the East belief that meditation has a very powerful way of making a pathway into the brain. We do know that when we learn to mind the body, we learn to mend the mind. When we got the self-help model into India it was looked upon as some kind of import from the British Raj, and looked at with suspicion. We had to indigenise it. The best way to do that was to bring about what a famous monk, who lived for forty years on the rivers of Khabi, called the marriage of the East and West: a blend of Western science – with all its beautiful data and information about how the discursive brain can contribute to the Kouri – with the right brain, the cellular consciousness, and learning to listen to the body. It's so essential that we learn to listen to the body, because in the East we believe that there is no chemical solution for chemical dependency, at least up to now, and that it's a human issue. Mother Teresa has this explanation. All our centres have been operated by her. Thirteen bishops made this commitment to us, and Kripa Foundation is the organization we have worked with. Mother Teresa's bias was this – basically a human being is beyond any reductionistic categories and we have to look holistically with a blend of mysticism and science to bring about the unique balance between the right brain and the left brain.

A: Ms Jane Wilson: In a place like Phoenix house, alternative therapies have come in (and this came in on the back of HIV). At that time mainstream medicine pooh-poohed us for getting money for reflexology, aromatherapy, acupuncture, etc., which was very difficult. I do know a colleague in Norway has been using acupuncture and are about to publish their results. So using these alternative medicines is having an impact on Hep C within this population. This is a fascinating finding but again we have to think how we can mainstream some of what used to be marginalised approaches or 'silly' approaches. They're very, very useful for this population. Because giving more pharmacology and more drugs sometimes just increases the problem.

A: Ms Anna Quigley: In terms of some of what we call the alternatives – acupuncture, etc., – some of the community sector groups have actually been using them for quite a while now and are finding them very beneficial.

Topic: Regional Issues and the Role of the Church

Q: Ms Rosemary Finane: What are the panel's opinions about the inequality of the responses to the drug problem between rural and urban centres throughout the country? Substances do exist obviously outside of Dublin, but opiates also exist, cocaine is becoming a bigger problem and we have poly-drug users. But I also want to ask the question: what role do you think the Church has to play outside of Dublin, particularly in more rural centres in Ireland? What is the role of the Church in prevention and intervention policies?

A: Ms Anna Quigley: There is a huge leadership role for the Church, and I think they need to look at how they can revise supports for developing that leadership role, because I think you can't ask someone to take a leadership role if they're not informed or aware on the issue. So that's part of the Church's role, to ensure that there is some way that priests locally can have access to information and support for themselves in dealing with those issues. Otherwise it's probably not realistic that they would do it. Again in rural areas people can be even more isolated, so there is a challenge for the Church in how they can provide support around that.

A: Minister Eoin Ryan: Regarding Dublin and rest of the country, the reason we are reviewing it is because we realise it is very Dublin- and Cork-based and that there is a problem right around the country. We certainly don't want the problems we've had in Dublin to spread right through other parts of the country, and that's why we're reviewing it and hopefully it will be a more country-based drug strategy. Not that we're going to take away a lot of the essential work that's been done in Dublin – hopefully we'll increase that, but hopefully we'll come up with a strategy that is more country friendly than we have had up to now.

A: Dr Des Corrigan: In relation to the Church's role, I'll just echo what Anna said: leadership, leadership, leadership, and making sure through boards of management that prevention programmes are brought into place among the schools under the control and management of the Church, so that in those areas where treatment facilities are needed, the Church does the hard thing and tries to lead from the front. We've had it politically from both Chris Flood and Eoin Ryan, they've been consistent in their view about communities' responsibility in this area. Unfortunately at local level it hasn't been; local politicians have been part of the problem and not part of the answer. I would like to think that the local church would be part of the answer rather than part of the problem.

Also, just in general, in terms of the urban versus rural, I'll just mention the fact that we need to take on board that there are different addictions. There are a whole range of drugs other than opiates and, even at European level, it is a struggle to get people not to be 'opio-centric', that is, just totally fixated on opiates and not seeing any other form of chemical problem developing, and I think we need to take that on board. I think the ASTI indicated a serious issue that we all need to worry about, because if our future is in the hands of young people, in an information society, those young people cannot be educated, no matter what class they come from, in a chemically impaired environment, and that's the challenge they face and that's the challenge we face. So I think it is an issue that can't just be divided between urban and rural; I think that urban–rural divide no longer exists, given the shape of this country and the speed at which one can move from city to town to countryside. I think it's an artificial divide.

Comment: Sr Kathleen Kelleher: I got so much out of today. I just wanted to correct one expression, and that was that there is a strategy for Dublin as opposed to the rest of the country; there's a strategy for parts of Dublin, but there is a lot of Dublin that isn't catered for.

CLOSING ADDRESS

Bishop Eamonn Walsh

Local Communities

Families and local communities have, and continue to be, the unsung heroes of the battle against drugs. After taking to the streets, they made everyone sit up and take heed. Quickly their focus shifted from 'Pushers Out', to getting treatment for those on street drugs and taking preventative steps that would enable the young to say 'No' to drugs. Parents and families were given hope and the Task Forces were established.

On behalf of the Bishops' Drugs Initiative Committee, I wish to publicly acknowledge all the community groups, many of whom are represented here today, for your courage, determination, genuine care and good common sense. Today is an attempt to provide a public platform for your current and future concerns. The theme of the *Beyond Maintenance* Seminar is what community groups have been asking to be resourced.

Maintenance – an intermediary step

Maintenance is intended as a step along the path of recovery rather than an indefinite ticking-over state of being. Used properly it can give time to reflect, to seek a new life-style, to catch up on delayed maturity and eventually to build up the necessary life-skills to become a responsible parent and constructive member of the community.

There is a growing tendency to leave people on long-term maintenance. In addition to the addictive nature of some drug substitutes and their many side effects, there is the danger that those on such maintenance can be forgotten because criminal activity to support drug habits has dropped. The social irritant factor has diminished and a public perception reassures that things are improving.

Holistic Treatment

A commitment is needed from statutory and voluntary bodies that maintenance for those who require it be short term and that those capable of natural detoxification methods are adequately catered for.

A holistic treatment for all who abuse drugs is where energies and resources are being called for. Within such treatment, underlying causes are addressed, lost years are recovered, self-esteem and pride are restored and a taste for life becomes real again.

Dignity for Everyone

All of this presumes that policy-makers and the wider community believe that drug users have hope in life and are capable of living as responsible and productive citizens.

Too often the language used to describe those on drugs betrays an attitude that they are 'no hopers'. This language can so easily percolate into public perceptions and expectations.

Drug users are not 'no hopers', they are not 'junkies', they are not 'low-lifes'. They are people born like you and me who have become entangled in a web of addictive living. They are in need of treatment that respects their inner potential and dignity. Treatment that will replace their distant glazed stare with life and ambition.

Waiting Lists

Most people are familiar with the difficulties in persuading someone who is abusing alcohol to agree to treatment. Imagine having struggled through intervention and persuasion to get him or her to avail of help only to be told, 'Come back in six weeks' or even 'six months'. Yet this is a daily frustration for family and friends of drug users. So often motivation cannot be maintained without help for weeks or months. Death sometimes intervenes. This is an urgent cry that so often goes unanswered in many areas.

Clear Message

Mixed messages about drugs are unhelpful at this time. Legislation of drugs is not the issue of the day. Real meaningful treatment is.

Words of Thanks

I would like to thank you all for coming here today and supporting this seminar. In a special way, on behalf of all present, may I thank our speakers and those who contributed from the floor: Archbishop Connell, Minister Eoin Ryan, Jim Cusack of *The Irish Times,* Anna Quigley of CityWide, Breda and Richie, Jane Wilson, Dr Des Corrigan and Chris Murphy.

I would also like to thank Monsignor Briscoe and the staff of Clonliffe College for the use of the College and catering, as well as the Organising Committee: Paula O'Gorman, Susan O'Neill, Peter O'Brien, Fr Paul Lavelle and all the members of the Bishops' Drugs Initiative Committee.

I thank Mr Conor Brady, Editor of *The Irish Times* for so readily agreeing to support and be associated with the seminar. This has been a twin-pulpit approach. Thank you all for being part of it.

APPENDIX

A FAITH RESPONSE TO THE STREET DRUG CULTURE

A Report from the Irish Centre for Faith and Culture

Eoin G. Cassidy

Introduction

In July 1999, in response to an invitation from Bishop Eamonn Walsh of the Irish Catholic Bishops' Drugs Initiative, the Irish Centre for Faith and Culture (ICFC), based in Maynooth, established a working party to explore 'a faith response to the street drug culture'. The group met from September '99 to June '00.

Two terms of reference were given particular priority, namely:

- Exploring the spirituality components in treatment and rehabilitation programmes, and promoting spirituality in programmes where it is not currently included;

- Gathering together the fruits of our listening to the spiritual life of heroin users.

The group was chaired by Joe Lucy, a Salesian priest who has spent many years in youth and community work in deprived areas of Dublin. For the past three years he has been director of Crinan, a programme based in the inner city of Dublin, whose aim is to rehabilitate young heroin users. The other members also brought to the working party a wealth of experience in academic, pastoral and other related fields. They were as follows: Joe Coyne PP, Patrick Doyle, Bernadette Flanagan PBVM, Pauline Logue IBVM, Tony MacCartaigh, Louise Monaghan, Maire O'Higgins, Tony O'Riordan SJ and Pauline Coughlan (secretary).

On behalf of the ICFC, it is appropriate for me to acknowledge the dedication and professionalism that characterized the voluntary contribution afforded by all the members to this project. Given their many work and/or family commitments, their willingness to participate in this initiative is particularly appreciated by the ICFC.

The ICFC was established in 1997 to foster an awareness of the complex relationship between faith and culture. In this context, it is of the first importance to acknowledge the extent to which the loss of self-esteem, occasioned by the lack of any sense of being loved by God or by one's fellow human beings, can contribute to creating a climate in which a drug culture can flourish. Similarly, one should be slow to underestimate the importance of nurturing the inner spiritual resources of those whose lives are marked by the human tragedy that is heroin abuse. In this light, I have no doubt that this report will make a significant contribution to our understanding of the importance of a faith response to the street drug culture, one that scars so much of our urban landscape.

Spirituality: Treatment and Rehabilitation Services

The first task that we set ourselves was to get a sense of the place of spirituality in existing services. This work was prompted by views expressed among our members that:

- Spirituality is a missing or underdeveloped component in most treatment and rehabilitation services.

- This absence is taking place in a culture of fading traditions where there is less and less attending to the spirit.

- People whose spirits are most visibly crushed by drug addiction are particularly needy of this kind of holistic support.

To this end, a brief questionnaire was prepared and sent to the directors of seventy-eight treatment and/or rehabilitation centres in the Republic of Ireland.[1] The purpose was to get a sense of whether or not centres had an explicit or even an implicit spirituality component on their programmes. The questionnaire also invited respondents to

indicate whether or not they were interested in fur
on the relationship between spirituality and
individual site visits were also organized. From ou.
conversations with people working in various drug treatment
and reflecting on our own experience, a number of points emerged.

- There is a wide degree of consensus that there is much room for improvement in delivering a 'holistic' treatment for drug addicts.

- Many of the gaps in services to people with drug addictions relate to very basic needs such as accommodation, access to medical models of treatment, counselling and detox services. Recommendations relating to increased provision and adequate standards in services are adequately expressed in the Irish Catholic Bishop's Policy Statement 1998, *Tackling Drug Problems Together*.

- Our survey and conversations also showed a high degree of consensus that, when it came to those aspects of helping the addict develop the 'power' within himself/herself to overcome addiction, nourishment of the spirit understood in a wide sense is seen as key, and yet many professionals felt that this area was largely underdeveloped for two reasons:

  1. The services in which they worked, as structured, didn't allow for much scope to develop this aspect of recovery.

  2. The professionals felt they needed support to deliver such aspects with confidence and many indicated that they would be interested in 'further conversations with us'.

In addition to the above, it seems to be the case that there is little evidence of the existence of an appropriate theoretical framework within which a spiritual response to drug addiction might be situated. The absence of such a framework is rendered more acute in the light of evidence that an over-association between spirituality and organised religion has led some to be reluctant to use the word spirituality in a

...lar context – especially in services funded by public monies. The ...ar is that the emphasis suggested by this approach will lead to ...ndoctrination into confessional religion. Although this interpretation is misplaced, the fears expressed need to be acknowledged.

In addressing these fears it can be helpful to express our spiritual heritage in easily accessible secular terms, such as 'self-esteem'. In religious terms, this may translate into knowledge that one is loved; one is created as a unique being and is called to be creative in the world and called uniquely.

Spirituality: Perspectives from Theory and Experience

Irrespective of the language used, the process in all cases is one of fundamental discovery by the individual that they have an inner life that can help them become freer persons – Christian spirituality seeks to free people and increase their freedom to choose to be people who more and more make things happen, rather than being people who powerlessly accept things that happen to them. In other words when we talk of spirituality, we are talking about behaviours and attitudes that are influenced by a sense of oneself that stems from inside.

A spirituality approach is process orientated and respectful of each person's story. As an approach, it is not one that requires a large commitment of effort into providing new resources. There are many suitable programmes that currently exist under the heading of personal development, self-esteem and empowerment programmes, etc. The challenge for people of faith, who believe that God's grace works through human tools, is to affirm people who use these tools. For people of faith whose primary training is in the use of these 'secular' tools, it is important to help them recognise the underlying spiritual dimension. This might be achieved by writing (a newsletter), or by workshops to help professionals who deliver these programmes to develop their own sense of the 'spiritual' nature of these programmes and to lobby for more holistic provision in drug treatment services.

A further challenge is to expand on this and offer aspects of our spiritual heritage that are not to be found within the secular helping programmes. This may include meditation, prayer (petitionary and contemplative), sacramental life of the Church, pilgrimage, etc.

The Oblate writer Ronald Rolheiser has developed some insights

into spirituality that are worthy of reflection[3] v
making a spiritual response to the street drug cul?
spoken of the misunderstandings that surround the te..
'chief among these is the idea that spirituality is, somehow,
esoteric and not something that issues forth from the bread and but..
of ordinary life…. Long before we do anything explicitly religious at
all, we have to do something about the fire that burns within us; what
we do with that fire, how we channel it, is our spirituality'[4].
Spirituality is more about whether or not we can sleep at night than
about whether or not we go to church. It is about being integrated or
falling apart, about being within community or being lonely. More
affirmatively, he has asserted that 'The opposite of being spiritual …
is to have no energy, is to have lost all zest for living – lying on a couch,
watching football or sitcoms, taking beer intravenously! But providing
us with energy is only half of the soul's job. Its other task, and a very
vital one it is, is to keep us glued together, integrated, so that we do
not fall apart and die'[5]. Under this aspect the opposite of a spiritual
person would be someone who has lost his or her identity, namely the
person who at a certain point does not know who he or she is
anymore. A healthy soul keeps both energised and glued together.[6]

A useful background to understanding spirituality and addiction
has been developed by the highly regarded psychologist of spirituality,
Gerald May. He has drawn attention to the fact that addiction to
drugs must be understood in the wider context of addictive living. In
other words, everybody struggles with addiction, whether it's to
security or ideas, substances or work. Addiction arises from the human
energy of desire getting attached and glued to something that is
perceived to meet the desire. Desire can also get attached to great
ideals of love and generosity. Gerald May has helpfully outlined how
the great wisdom traditions of the world have all reflected on how to
achieve freedom of desire (detachment), which of course is not
freedom from desire.[7] One example from the wisdom of the past is the
Greek philosopher Heraclitus who observed that the need for
attachment is often fulfilled 'at the cost of the soul'.

The Dublin urban theologian Martin Byrne has noted that context
and culture are also significant factors to consider when seeking to
understand a specific spirituality. He defines *contextual spirituality* as

ocusing of spiritual reflection from a particular localised situation ich gives a definite perspective and flavour to the project. Cultural dentity, social change and popular religiosity are taken into consideration along with the elements of scripture and tradition'[8]. He also offers a definition of culture as 'the concrete context in which life happens. It represents a way of life for a given time and place, replete with values, symbols and meanings, reaching out with hopes and dreams, often struggling for a better world'[9].

The Stories

As well as offering a theoretical framework for recommending a spiritual response to the street drug culture, we also undertook to gather reflections on spirituality from heroin users in order to ground the theory in reality. The reflections below are drawn from the collated responses of interviews with four men and four women, who were mostly in their twenties.[10] The aim is first of all to itemise, in a more detailed fashioned, specific issues that will shape any spiritual response. The second task is to outline a general spiritual response to the street drug culture by drawing parallels between comments in the interviews and the Emmaus story.[11]

Frances's Story

I'm twenty-three. I have four brothers and one sister. A couple of them take drugs, I'm on a methadone programme myself and my mother and father. My father and mother were chronic alcoholics and thank God he is off it a year and a half now and she is off it for the last three years. The rest of the family are great at supporting us because of the programmes we're on. I'm out looking for a job now. I've actually got a job appointment this morning and I hope to get that job.

All my family used to take drugs and now there are only three of us left on methadone programmes. It has really changed now from what it was like back then. It was hassle all the time, constant trouble, whether it was over drugs, drink, what you'd be wearing in the house or family rows. We're now stable on the methadone programme and hopefully we'll all do well and next year we'll be able to say that we're all clean.

I was on drugs for about seven years from about the age of fourteen to twenty-one. The toughest time for myself was having to go out and rob and take things from people. I knew I was hurting them and their family but I needed the money and that was just the way it was. I didn't care who I was taking it from or who I hurt or anything. I didn't think of my family, I was just thinking of my fix and getting my fix into me, I didn't care about anybody else, my mother, my father or anybody else. I thought at the time that I was just going through a phase. I was taking a bit of heroin and thought that I could take it or leave it, but a couple of months later things were very different. One morning, I was really sick. I just thought I had the flu but it wasn't the flu and I had to be put on a methadone programme and I was saying 'Oh God, what am I going to do?' At that time I felt suicidal, I slit my wrists and was signed into hospital.

I didn't really think there was a God then because I was saying that if there was a God, this wouldn't have happened to me. Through all the years of pain and suffering I went through I was saying, 'There couldn't be a God up there. He's not even helping me'. I tried so many times to come off the stuff and I couldn't come off it. When I hit the age of eighteen I got myself into a detox programme and after I was clean for nearly a year, I started believing there was a God there. It was just a matter of time before he came to me. It is just a matter of time before he comes to everyone.

How would I describe how it was? I was getting the love and care that I had missed. I was making friends, I was going out meeting new people, going to things like NA meetings and things that I would never have done and now I believe there is a God.

He's in my heart and I do believe in God now. I've good belief in God. I never went to Mass and now I go to Mass. The last time I ever went to Mass was for my confirmation. Now I go on Sundays, even if its only for half an hour, I go to say prayers for a few friends and pray for myself to help me that day, that's how much it's changed me. When I go to Mass, it's actually very important. I go to Mass because there is a God, before I didn't believe in him but he was always there. As I've got older and wiser I have begun to believe that no matter what you believe or do, he will help you.

When I go into Mass now I feel a great relief and I can talk to the priest and tell him all my sins. I know he listens to me and doesn't criticise me. He just tells me to go and say a few Hail Marys. I feel accepted.

Jesus wouldn't actually have a meaning for me except that I go into Mass and I see him up on the cross, nailed to the cross. My father used to tell me that he had to drag that over his shoulder and they nailed him to the cross. I couldn't believe it when they told me all this. I said this couldn't be true. Now when I go into church I kneel down in front of him and I always say a prayer. I don't say 'Dear God', I always say 'Dear Jesus' because of what he went through, because it must have been very hard for him.

I remember my confirmation day – I had a great day. Before confirmation we all went to confession and the priest said I was forgiven and I felt brilliant. He was helping me and he said that Jesus had forgiven me for what I'd done. I'd just to go out and say a few prayers so I went out and said a few prayers. It was great, all that day I wasn't thinking about my confirmation, I was thinking about what happened that morning and to me it was brilliant – even now.

To me church is for going to Mass, and I do go to Mass. I like priests. I actually get on with some of them very well. I say a prayer every night before I go to bed. I pray for myself, my family and friends I've lost. I say a prayer and hope that I'll wake up in the morning.

I've had a very bad experience of going through drugs. I was backed into a corner probably like other addicts are now and thought I would never get out. I'd advise them to go to counselling because no matter what you say it is kept private. If you hold everything back, because you think people are going to laugh at you, you're probably paranoid. The counselling is actually very good. I'd also advise them to go to healing groups and massages, join in drama groups, go to family centres and other support groups. It really does help.

How would I describe myself? Well, I'm actually a real nice person. I have a real soft heart. I probably try to put on an image now and again but that was when I was on drugs. I was trying to put on an image of something that I wasn't but I'm real soft and I'd do anything for anyone. One of my friends left me two years ago, we had an argument and now she's back with me again because she knows I'm a good friend. I wouldn't hold a grudge. I'd describe myself as an outgoing person, enjoying life and doing drama.

Dereck's Story

I'm twenty-five and I've been having serious trouble with heroin and cocaine for about three years. I've been in treatment for the past five weeks, three weeks in a clinic and five weeks clean.

I do pray. I say prayers for the kids and for Jenny, for God to make sure that they are alright and to take care of everyone in the house. I pray every night, every single night before I go to sleep. I can't go to sleep unless I do. I used to talk to God when I was small and I never really lost belief in him totally. I remember everything important when I was a kid. I remember talking to him, asking him to make all the stuff that was happening to me stop and to get me out of the situations I was in.

I wanted God to move me somewhere else – to live with some other people. I was asking God to protect me and he never did. After a while I felt like it was happening to me for a reason. When all these terrible things happened to me I felt that I must have done something horrible that I was being punished for by God. I just used to ask him for help but every family I was sent to abused me in some way or another. It happened everywhere, you tell me, you work it out for yourself. You constantly ask for help because you have no one else to talk to, and it just keeps happening. God is meant to be protecting you in some way or another, that's what you believe when you are a kid, only to find out He wasn't there for me.

Still, I do believe in him and I've been talking to him over the years. Bad things happen for a reason I suppose, I don't know what reason, but if I hadn't been in certain situations I wouldn't have met Jenny. There are parts of my life that I don't want to change.

I keep going back to when I was a kid, I am sort of stuck in that. I'm sure there were one or two nice things too but I can't remember them. The bad outweighed the good. I'd no trust in anybody, I used to run away from the children's home. I couldn't stay in one place for longer than a couple of weeks and then I'd have to move on, that's just the way I got, I used to run all the time.

I couldn't trust God because I'd seen the Church as part of God and they abused me. This was the Church, with so-called agents of God having an agenda that wasn't a good one, so what belief could you have? When you see that, belief in normal people, I mean people who aren't priests, goes out the window. Priests and people of the Church are always portrayed as good people and there are some who can sit and talk and give you a little bit of belief and hope, but then all that is taken away as well.

Still, I do pray to God at night, I ask him to look after everybody and thank him for looking after me. But it's only recently I thank him for looking after me, before I never did, it was just for everyone else. In a way I felt it wasn't right to ask God to look after you when you were saying prayers, it was kind of a selfish thing to do. I felt I should ask him to look after other people and people who were dead.

I thank him for helping me get through yesterday because I'm having a rough time. I know he's helping me for not using when I feel like using or when I get depressed and then I ask him to help me get through today and I think he does. I think something must be going right for me.

Always when I walk by a church I bless myself because you never know what's down the road. I also bless myself when I see an ambulance because it could be rushing for someone you know. If you bless yourself it's like saying a little prayer hoping that they'll get to the person in time. It's like wishing them goodwill.

Funerals and weddings in church is the right thing to do, it's the proper way to do it. I hope that when my kids get married, if they decide to, that that's what they'll do. It's not just that it's the place to get married, it's sacred. I'd like to bring the kids to church. I don't know why I don't. I used to go to church every Sunday when I was a kid and I used to love listening to the stories out of the Bible. It's a long time since I've been to church and part of it is I'm afraid I mightn't know when to sit down, stand up and kneel down properly. Sometimes when I pass by a church I go in and light candles, when I'm worried about somebody or something and I feel I really need something, I go in and light a couple of candles. I just pray that Jenny and the kids are alright, that they're safe during the day. That's all I pray for, you know.

Eamon's Story
Life is miserable, I don't even know why I carry on. I wouldn't care if I got smacked by a bus tomorrow, it wouldn't bother me. There's no magic pill that you can just take. I just carry on. I rarely have good times

but when I had my twins around, then times were good. That was about two years ago. I just move on, I don't know what keeps me going but I'm doing good off the drugs, I'm on the methadone. I don't go near the heroin, I don't go near stuff like that. They just give me some methadone every day and that keeps me going, keeps me away from stealing. I do have a few quid now and again because I'm not spending it on drugs. I think everybody who's on gear should be given a free course because they're the only ones really stealing. When you see cars flying around they're just teenagers, you know fourteen- to fifteen-year-olds, they're not on drugs. They're just messers who'll end up on the gear.

I believe in heaven. Maybe that's the reason why I'm not afraid to die. Heaven is not a place where you're going to meet people, it's a peaceful place. It's like a baby in its mother's womb, nice and peaceful, happy as Larry. Whereas the other place people call hell, you meet the devil, you're not in a peaceful place, you're in a horrible place.

I don't feel any kind of link with God or Jesus and I don't pray but I believe in God and I believe in Jesus. It's the Mary bit and the Immaculate Conception that's a bit far-fetched and it's not fair on Joseph, is it! When I was in prison, I used to go to Mass every Sunday. Some priests are great at giving out Mass, some priests just want to get it over and done with. People would leave and say Jesus, that's the last time I'm going there. Some priests would really be very good giving out Mass and people would go again to hear him. You suss that out when you are in prison.

I got off drugs when I got onto a course. I was determined not to get back into that life again. Heroin is an evil drug, sent from an evil source. It really is. It's like the devil controls your life. You do the most horrible things, like stealing, you don't care who you rob.

I think the spark that keeps me going is that I know there is a worse place. Where I am today, I know there is a place a million times worse. If I start messing around with heroin, I know where I'm going to end up and that's the spark that keeps me going. Methadone is the magical drug. Magical. You don't get stoned on it and it keeps you stable. Nobody would know you were on heroin. Well, I'm not on heroin now, I'm on methadone. I think that if everyone was put onto methadone, the drug dealers would go out of business. Heroin would be gone. I mean it.

When I was growing up, I used to love my religion. I wouldn't rob because it was a sin. I was a good child, because I really thought that when you sinned, God was looking at you. It's like as if you clocked up so many sins, you'd go to hell. I don't want to go to hell and that is the main reason. People nowadays are evil. They're all out for themselves. People are bad, they'd stab you in the back. Everyone's robbing and shooting each other, and politicians and even priests and Christian Brothers; everything has blown up in Irish people's faces.

I always got on great with children. When we had only one child, it was me who got up at six in the morning to get that bottle. I was more the Mammy than anything else. When it came to the twins, it was more her. The children were the best things that ever happened to me. I think they are what keep me going. I think they are the best things that happened in my life. It's brilliant to see them grow, they're learning all the time and love watching everything. You could be talking and wouldn't even know they're listening and then they turn around and say, 'Say that again'. It's amazing. They keep me going.

I never really looked inside myself but I know that inside I'm a really good person. I'd prefer everybody to be nice, honest and to get on with each other. There are a lot of rotten people out there. Why did they crucify Him, why did they nail Him to the cross? My son, he's six now and when he asks me why, it's very hard to explain it to him.

I'd like the kids to go to church because then they'd have a direction in life. If they don't go to Mass, they've nothing. I think the church is what keeps people sane. It makes people think twice about doing horrible things. I don't really have the time to go to Mass myself but I do have holy medals and pictures. I have loads of them and I have them all over my room. They mean a lot to me because when the young fella stays with me he sees them and asks me about them. So I tell him. He always blesses himself going by the church. One day he asked me why I didn't bring him to church and I told him to wait until he made his First Holy Communion and then he could go to church. He thought it was wrong not to go to church. He's a pure innocent, you know.

Noreen's Story
The baby keeps me going. He's brought a whole new thing into my

life. He could have died when he was born, I could have died myself. The baby pulled through and everything was great. I felt there was someone watching over us. It was through the pregnancy and when the baby was born that I began to feel that there was somebody there, before that, I didn't really feel it as strongly.

The day I found out that I was pregnant, I found this little relic. It's a little cloth and on the back of it, it says 'St Anthony – cloth touched to relic of St Anthony whom the Infant loved and honoured, obtain for us what we ask of thee'. Now some people can make loads out of that and that could have been the Infant Jesus, but to me that made out it was my infant and I always kept that with me, 'obtain for us what myself and Harry ask of the Lord'. I always felt that and I have always kept it with me. The baby's bag, it was always in the baby's bag. The very day I found out that I was pregnant, I was walking down O'Connell St, we had just come from the family planning clinic and it was actually lashing rain. I picked the relic up and I said to Harry 'Look at that', I was reading it and I said 'Look at that'. Some people say it's good luck to find holy medals and some people say it's bad luck, but I think it was good luck to find it. I think maybe it was meant for me to find it.

When the baby was sick, I knew my Grandda wouldn't let anything happen to him or my friends that had died. I just prayed to whoever was up there. I just kept praying and hoping. I was just praying that whoever is up there, please, just please look after Edward, and they did. I just know that there is somebody there, I don't know who it is. At that time I had a drug problem. Well, I'm still on methadone but I have my ups and downs as everyone does, but I always pull through for the baby's sake. Someone is always asking me what's going to happen to the baby if I go down that road again.

I know it's very selfish but I only pray when I want something, or when I need something. Before the baby was born, if I didn't get what I wanted I'd say, there's no God up there. But now I really pray, I'd bless myself when going past a church or a funeral. I don't pray every night but the nights I do pray, I pray for something that I want. I say a decade of the Rosary. I don't think there is hell there but there is evil. There is an evil side in everyone and the evil side in me sometimes stops me from praying. Even when I went to confession years ago, bless me Father for I have sinned and then I wouldn't know what to say. You know when the priest says, 'what are your sins?' in confession – still to this day the only thing I'm able to say is, 'I was cursing to me Ma and Da'. It's like when I was in school.

After things worked out with the baby, I thanked God. I didn't know who to thank but I was praying, I just said, 'thank you whoever is up there, thanks very much for everything that's working out'. I didn't know who to actually pray to. You know the way people have a saint that they pray to, well, some nights I'd be lying in bed and I'd pray to St Anthony or St Martin – you know, Harry's brother's name was Martin.

The low point in my life was when I was in prison. I slit my wrists, I just wanted to end it all, but there was always somebody there for me, like my family, I didn't want to hurt them too much. Now I have a new life with Harry and he keeps me going as well. Before that it was just a struggle to get what I needed – find a place to stay, get money, get drugs, that's all I really thought about to be quite honest. There was always a lot of guilt there, even when I was on drugs. Anything I did I always felt bad about it. I think there's a lot of guilt inside me. I always knew I shouldn't be taking drugs. I was always saying every day I have to get myself together. I used to say to God if I had a little baby I'd get myself off drugs.

When I met Harry first we weren't in love, we were just a drug couple. Then both of us got locked up and then I think we started thinking what we meant to each other. On my side anyway, I started thinking what he meant to me and what we went through together. When I was out of my house, he had a home to go to but he stayed out on the street with me because he wouldn't leave me on my own. He had enough for drugs and he could have just said he was going home to bed. He never once left me out on the street on my own. That's one thing that I like about him, you know. I admire him for it, he was always there for me.

I just knew that taking drugs was wrong. When I was young, my mother would be watching the news and something bad would come on and they'd talk about it then and I'd know it was wrong to do. I actually used to look down on people using drugs, I used to think they were scum using that stuff and then when I tried it meself, I thought it's just like people make it out to be. You know, I didn't think I could go down so low, but I did.

I know there's a lot of people there for me. I have my family back now and I have a lot of people there for me. If I want to talk to anyone, there are loads of people I can talk to. It's just that I know I'm not on my own any more. I've loads of support if I need it. The baby is just everything to me. He is, he's just everything to me.

Mary's Story

I'm twenty-three, single and live with my mother and three brothers. I've been on drugs since I was sisteen. I suppose my mother is very religious, I'm not very religious myself because God shouldn't have let me have the life I had when I was a child. It was hard and it still is hard. My father hit me all the time, he was an alcoholic. Then I lost three kids in a miscarriage. I had a nervous breakdown, I just snapped, I couldn't take any more of it, then after that I got bad news that I had got HIV. I'm not really coping well, I'm not really coping at all. I just feel depressed all the time.

I remember my First Holy Communion day and my Confirmation day. They were good days. My mother, my granny – almost all the family were there. My father never came because he just had a grudge against me. I don't know why.

I believed in God at one stage, I still do a bit. I know there is somebody there, there has to be somebody there, but why does God put you in this world to be hurt? I can't stand people hurting each other, messing their whole lives up.

Sometimes I pray when I'm on my own. I ask for help, for one thing – to help me to have a child. That's my wish. If that happened to me, I'd believe there was a God because then he was listening to me. I did pray and I used to wish all the hurt would stop. I couldn't cope at all. I was the oldest at the time, I was seven, but I still remember and I'm going back trying to get it all out of my head. My mother, she doesn't understand, I was only a child but I still remember everything. She says to just ignore it but I can't ignore it, it won't leave my head. Loads of things won't leave my head. Even today, these things are holding me down.

I pray to God even though I see God as a blur. I pray to the Virgin

Mary for help, to give me a chance. I know I did a lot of bad stuff but I'm sorry for doing what I did. I've been out of trouble for years, it's just that I went off the rails a bit that's all, that's all this mess.

Nowadays some people don't go to Mass, but they do pray in their own way. I don't go to Mass but sometimes I do pray when I need a little help to help me get through this day or something is on my mind, but I don't need priests. Now my mother, she's real religious, she goes to Mass, she reads the bible and she's trying to get me to read it too. There can be a lot of hypocrisy in religion – people stab you in the back and then go to Mass. I used to go to Mass but I just stopped. I went to the Born-Again-Christians in England. Well, they would talk to you and explain things to you.

I think a lot about death. I'm afraid to die, I'm afraid of the pain, if I was going through pain, I would just want them to pull the plug on me and let me die. I wonder where I'm going. I wonder if there is a God. I wonder if I will see God.

Life is real short, you don't know when you are going to go. I would hope to have a child and have my own place and to enjoy my life when I can. I would like to get away from this area and if there is a God, he should listen to people and help people.

Jack's Story
I'm nineteen at the minute, I was fourteen when I started taking heroin. At the age of twelve I started drinking and started smoking hash and at the age of fourteen I started taking Es and then started on heroin.

I believe there is a God out there. I don't pray before I go to bed, but if I really am going through pain or emotional things, I would talk to him. Sometimes when I pray to God, it's about the drug use and to heal me. I do believe in him, I know there is a God there.

I felt special when I was in recovery. I prayed, I went to church and I thanked God that I'm still alive and I'm doing well and that. My mind was much clearer at that time. Drugs, you don't think about pain, you don't think of anything really, you just think about your next fix. The emotions are not there, it takes away your feelings. When I was on the programme and doing well, my head was much clearer but I did pray and I did pray that everything would be alright and for my mother and father.

I don't really go to church often, just once in a blue moon. If I'm feeling down or if I feel that something has to be changed or if I need help that's when I go down to the church. All I can do is hope.

I always wondered about heaven and about angels. I think heaven is a real peaceful place. The way I think of heaven is that everyone walks around in white gowns and everyone is friendly to each other. If there is a heaven, there also has to be a hell – good and evil, you know what I mean. I don't know whether to believe in it or not. I'm only going by what people say on the telly but you don't know till you die what happens.

Belinda's Story

I'm forty-three and I've three children, the eldest is twenty-two, the next is ten and the youngest is seven. I'm from the south inner-city and I have been involved with drugs over a good number of years.

I remember my First Holy Communion. It was frightening. Yeah, frightening. I remember my first confession, we were terrified going to the church. At that time, I was eight. Most of the others were about six or seven but I had been sick for a number of years. We were all terrified to go into confession. We didn't know what it was really and at that time there was the Latin Mass so we didn't really understand anything.

I went to a convent school. The nuns used to wear the long black habits, they were way above us and we were terrified of them, we were also terrified of the priests. We were brought up to fear them. There was a young priest that I got to know when I was very young and I could talk to him. He was more of a family friend and then down through the years a number of things happened and it didn't turn out too well for him in the end. That really I suppose turned me against priests. Looking back over the years, I suppose I blanked things out till they came and asked me about him.

I hope that God is there, I would like to think that he is. Sometimes I feel he is, other times I don't, but at the back of my mind I think there is somebody there. When things are going wrong, you say to yourself, if he is really there, how could he put me through this much? Down through life the way things went for me, every time I was up I got knocked back down. Going back to when I was a teenager, I had problems but I got over them. I got married. I did everything by the book, got engaged, saved, had a big wedding, put a deposit on a house, went back to work, sold the small house and bought a bigger one. When the first boy came along I gave up work, stayed at home and minded him. Everything ran smoothly for a few years. Then my husband started going wrong, he turned violent and that, that knocked me back a lot and I left him after a number of years. After that I tried to get up on my feet and make a go of it on my own, then I'd go back to him. I'm not doing anything wrong, I'm trying my best to bring up my kids.

The odd morning, on the way back from school, I might drop in and catch the end of Mass. When I'd come out of the church I'd always feel good. Even if I'd been in church for only ten minutes, I felt something. I had a contented feeling and I thought I'd go to Mass again because I like the feeling, a warm close kind of feeling and then you feel there is somebody there.

A church to me is just the building, just a big place, cold, that's usually what comes to mind. There has been over the years one or two priests I could talk to, but then again being brought up the way I was, I'd fear them. There is a lot of fear there still once you see the collar, but I think that nowadays the way a lot of priests dress just normal, I think that does help.

When I'm lying in bed on my own and things are really going bad, then I pray, not really prayers, just talking to God. I wonder how long more this is going to go on and if God can sort something out. To me prayer is not something you read out of a prayer book; it's just talking. For me now, Mass is a good thing. What comes to mind is that nice contented feeling but then again if I'm getting that contented feeling, I don't know why I don't make an effort and go to Mass more often. I suppose that when I just go by chance, I get that nice feeling.

It's the kids that keep me going, when the little fella says something, I'd just come over, put him on my lap and give him a hug. The days when I'm really in despair and something like that happens, it cheers me up. I'd love to just get a home and settle down and continue the way we are. We are a close family but I'd like to bring the smaller two up a bit better, with more in their life – in a lot of ways now, like religion. The ten-year-old asks me a lot about religion, like Mass and why we don't go. I just explain to her how I feel about Mass. She actually came a few times and likes going. A friend of mine brings her to Mass on a regular basis. Looking back when I was growing up, we went to 11.30 Mass every Sunday morning. It was a nice feeling and you met the aunts and uncles outside the church. I'd like something like that for them. When they are older they can make their own decision. I think it's important that you introduce them to it.

When I was growing up, everyone believed in heaven and hell. Now I can't see so clearly how some can go to heaven and others to hell, especially when I dwell on the life I had growing up, a lot of it was like going to hell. I can't understand why I went through what I did, but I don't think I was ever bad enough to deserve what I went through and that afterwards I might be punished again in hell.

I suppose that there is a God who created things years and years ago and that he has left his spirit behind for us, but at the end of the day, I can't see where we are going. I picture Jesus looking down, dressed in white with long hair, that's what flashes through my mind when I think of Jesus.

There are times when I look at the kids and wonder what is going to happen from here on. Is God there and is he going to make things easier for them? I feel that at Mass there has to be somebody there, then I just go on about the day and it just goes out of my mind.

I suppose I'm still searching, I suppose I'm hoping that somebody will say something to me someday and I will say, 'That's it'.

Hugh's Story

I'm now twenty but I started taking drugs when I was about fourteen. I was into drugs serious by the time I was fifteen. I started drinking first but I never really enjoyed drinking – I still don't really – and then I started smoking hash and going raving and taking Es and that led to the heroin.

I like the yoga with Miriam. It gets me in touch with part of me that I don't really know. It's something that I never thought I'd be able to do, to train my head and just meditate and relax. That's different.

Sometimes God comes into my mind, like before I go to bed at night I say a few prayers. I pray for my family and friends. I hope they're okay and nothing really bad happens. When I'm praying for my family I wish them well and hopefully myself too – so that I get over my drug addiction.

Well, when I was younger, before I took drugs, I used to go to Mass nearly every week. In the last few years, I haven't gone to Mass at all, only a few times but not as often as I should – not the normal Mass service. But I go to the Mass services for the people that died, yeah, but the normal, ordinary Mass, I haven't been to one of them for three or four years, except probably at Christmas. I used to go once a week, but when I got into the drugs I just lost interest. I lost interest in everything, my hobbies, a lot of things that I liked doing, like football. All I really cared about was taking drugs.

Church is a place where you go to pray whether it's for the people around you that you love or the people who are dying, it's just a place where you can go and have time for yourself and pray and speak your thoughts.

Recurring Themes

1.   The spirituality in the interviews was *community-based.* Prayer would refer to the family, to others in the community and to the dead: 'I say prayers for the kids, for Jenny, for God to make sure they are alright and to take care of everyone in the house' (Dereck). 'When my baby was sick I knew my Grandda wouldn't let anything happen to him, or my friends that had died. I just prayed to whoever was up there (in heaven)' (Noreen).

2.   *An inability to feel loved unconditionally by God* could reflect the lack of access to opportunities for development beyond a super-ego-based relationship with God: 'When all these terrible things happened to me I felt that I must have done something horrible that I was being punished for by God' (Dereck). 'You know when the priest says "What are your sins?" in confession. Still to this day the only thing I'm able to say is, "I was cursing me Ma and Da". It's like when I was in school' (Noreen).

3.   The spirituality of the interviewees was *survival-based* and told of a struggle for life in the face of overwhelming odds: 'Through all the years of pain and suffering I went through I was saying, "There couldn't be a God up there. He's not even helping me". I tried so many times to come off the stuff and I couldn't come

off it. When I hit the age of eighteen I got myself into a detox programme and after I was clean for nearly a year, I started believing there was a God there. It was just a matter of time before he came to me' (Frances).

4. *Children had a central place* in activating a sense of hope and desire for life amongst those interviewed: 'When we had only one child, it was me who got up at six in the morning to give him the bottle. I was more the Mammy than anything else' (Eamon). 'It was through the pregnancy and when the baby was born that I began to feel that there was somebody there, before that, I didn't really feel it as strongly' (Noreen).

5. Many comments on religion displayed a *humour* in the face of perceived absurdity *and an intolerance of hypocrisy:* 'I believe in God. I believe in Jesus. It's the Mary bit and the Immaculate Conception that's a bit far-fetched. And it's not fair on Joseph, is it!' (Eamon). 'There can be a lot of hypocrisy in religion – people stab you in the back and then go to Mass' (Mary).

6. Occasional glimpses of a *private devotional faith.*

BELINDA	————
FRANCES	The Crucifix
MARY	The Virgin Mary
NOREEN	St Anthony relic, The Rosary
DERECK	Light candles
EAMON	Religious medals, holy pictures crucifixes, the Devil
HUGH	————
JACK	Angels

7. The theme of *resistance* was strong in the conversations. Spirituality, therefore, needs to be consistent with developing a

fighting spirit and with the insistence on a better future. Mary, who was living with HIV, clearly defined her dreams for her future: 'I would hope to have a child, to have my own place and enjoy my life while I can, to get away from this area'.

8.   *Prayer* was a familiar spiritual practice in the lives of most of the interviewees and their comments generally echoed Belinda's view: 'To me prayer is not something you read out of a prayer-book; it's just talking'.

9.   Often a *sense of shame or alienation* infused the sense of not having the right to be in the Church. There were also *feelings of being awkward and uncomfortable in holy places*. 'When I dwell on the life I had growing up, a lot of it was like going to hell…. but I don't think I was ever bad enough to deserve what I went through and that afterwards I might be punished again in hell' (Belinda). 'It's a long time since I've been to church and part of it is I'm afraid I mightn't know when to sit down, stand up and kneel down properly' (Dereck).

10. A tension *between spirituality and religion* was evident in some of the comments: 'Nowadays some people don't go to Mass, but they do pray in their own way' (Mary).

11. Contact with *new structures for supporting interiority and spirituality* were also evident in the lives of some of those interviewed: Born-Again Church (Mary), counselling, drama, healing, massage, support groups (Frances), yoga (Hugh).

12. *The experience of religion was ambiguous.* Some comments revealed how the experience of Church and the experience of God were intertwined negatively: 'I couldn't trust God because I'd seen the Church as part of God and they abused me' (Dereck). Mary pointed out that it was easier to have a sense of God in the Born-Again Church because 'they would talk to you and explain things to you'.

Much has been said everywhere about the decline of religious belief; not so much notice has been taken of the decline of religious sensibility. The trouble of the modern age is not merely the inability to believe certain things about God and man, which our forefathers believed, but the inability to feel towards God and man as they did.[12]

Echoing T. S. Eliot then, it seems to emerge from the comments above that it is not simply a case of religion being dead or dormant in the lives of those who live with addiction, but rather that they feel about religion in a new way.

Heroin and the Holy: When Strangers Meet

People nowadays are evil. They're all out for themselves. People are bad, they'd stab you in the back. Everyone's robbing and shooting each other, and politicians and even priests and Christian Brothers; everything has blown up in Irish people's faces (Eamon).

My father hit me all the time, he was an alcoholic. Then I lost three kids in a miscarriage. I had a nervous breakdown, I just snapped, I couldn't take any more of it, then after that I got bad news that I had got HIV. I'm not really coping well, I'm not really coping at all. I just feel depressed all the time.... I believed in God at one stage, I still do a bit. I know there is somebody there, there has to be somebody there, but why does God put you in this world to be hurt? I can't stand people hurting each other, messing their whole lives up.... I did pray and I used to wish all the hurt would stop. I couldn't cope at all. I was the oldest at the time, I was seven, but I still remember and I'm going back trying to get it all out of my head. My mother, she doesn't understand, I was only a child but I still remember everything. She says to just ignore it but I can't ignore it, it won't leave my head. Loads of things won't leave my head. Even today, these things are holding me down.... If there is a God he should listen to people and help people (Mary).

In our study group we were looking at what might be a spiritual response to the street drug culture. From the two snippets of conversation above, which were part of interviews with drug users on their experience of religion and spirituality, it is clear that the current level of addiction may need to be understood against the current cultural background. Forms of pain and sorrow that were once hidden are now in the public forum. It isn't possible to ignore darker aspects of life that were previously more secret. Those persons and institutions that once inspired public confidence and provided an anchor of security have been found to be unreliable and frail. This is provoking confusion, uncertainty, disillusionment and mistrust on a grand scale.

Let us walk together

Luke's story of the two disciples on the road to Emmaus (Lk 23:13-35) may be being played out on the streets of Irish cities and towns today. Like the disciples in the Lucan story, those interviewed in our survey spoke freely about their lives, their struggles, their questions and their hopes. They too were questioning where God was in their story. They had, for the most part, turned their backs on the old Jerusalem, the securities of their First Communion and Confirmation faith. None however had reached Emmaus. In other words, while they were clear about leaving what had been, there was a lack of clarity about what could be believed in. This was particularly evident in the searching for a way to name God: 'Whoever is up there (Heaven), please look after Edward' (Noreen).

Are we listening?

Like the disciples on the road to Emmaus, the interviewees had a great desire to make sense of the confusion in their lives. For this reason, conversational interventions were particularly welcomed: 'there are good people in the Church who can sit and talk and give you a little bit of belief and a little bit of hope' (Dereck). This echoes the experience of which Jean Vanier spoke in his book *Becoming Human*.[13] In that book he observed that listening tells another 'You are important. Your whole being, your experiences, opinions and observations matter'. Listening is experienced as the embodied fulfilment of the Christian call to love the neighbour. Listening is the ground from which experiences of growth, healing and reorientation may emerge.

How will we respond?

In general it was evident in the interviews that religious vocabulary was limited: 'Some priests are great at giving out Mass' (Eamon). Contact with the formal expressions of religion were also rare: 'I go to Mass services for the people who die – but the normal ordinary Mass, I haven't been to one of them for three or four years, except probably at Christmas' (Hugh). However, like the Emmaus disciples, the interviewees often welcomed an introduction to religious practices and images even though they were unfamiliar with them: 'Yoga is something that I thought I'd never be able to do, to train my head and just to meditate and relax. That's different' (Hugh). A latent hunger for the spiritual is available to be awakened. There is an interest in the skills of interiority, 'I never really looked inside myself' (Eamon).

Do not underestimate love made flesh

For the Emmaus disciples, the meal was a pivotal moment of recognition. No longer were they simply talking about their hopes and fears with the stranger, they were now embodying forth a shared world of meaning. In the passing around of food, the experience of solidarity of conviction on the road was transformed into a solidarity of sharing. In the experience of breaking bread with the stranger, it was recognised that Love was present. The interviewees also witnessed to the powerful impact of embodied solidarity on their lives: 'When I met Harry first we weren't in love, we were just a drug couple. Then both of us got locked up and then I think we started thinking what we meant to each other. On my side anyway, I started thinking what he meant to me and what we went through together. When I was out of my house, he had a home to go to but he stayed out on the street with me because he wouldn't leave me on my own. He had enough for drugs and he could have just said he was going home to bed. He never once left me out on the street on my own. That's one thing that I like about him, you know. I admire him for it, he was always there for me' (Noreen). An incipient conviction about the place of community in the living of a fully human life seems to be evident in this story.

Recognising the grace at work in addiction

Just as the two disciples were empowered by their Emmaus encounter, so also it is evident that the seeds for renewal may be present in the experience of those who live with addiction for those who have eyes to see. The challenge, which those interviewed raised consistently, is the possibility of the experience of a this-worldly fullness of life as an experience of Christian faith. Put another way, while conversation about God is not deemed impossible, the experience of God is fragile: 'I'm not very religious myself because God shouldn't have let me have the life I had when I was a child. It was hard and it still is hard' (Mary). In the spirituality of the future it will not be possible, it seems, to bypass the suffering of the world in the journey to God. Indeed, it was interesting that it was the image of the innocent suffering Christ that spoke to Frances: 'Jesus wouldn't actually have a meaning for me except that I go into Mass and I see him up on the cross, nailed to the cross. My father used to tell me that he had to drag that over his shoulder and they nailed him to the cross. I couldn't believe it when they told me all this. I said this couldn't be true. Now when I go into church I kneel down in front of him and I always say a prayer. I don't say 'Dear God', I always say 'Dear Jesus' because of what he went through, because it must have been very hard for him.'

The Emmaus story seems then to provide a model for approaching the question of finding a spiritual response to the street drug culture.

Notes

1. As listed in *The Treatment and Rehabilitation Directory* (The Department of Health, 1999).
2. See 'Response to the Short Questionnaire' on page 94.
3. R. Rolheiser, *Seeking Spirituality: Guidelines for a Christian Spirituality for the Twenty-First Century* (London: Hodder & Stoughton, 1998).
4. Ibid., p. 6.
5. Ibid., p. 11.
6. Ibid.
7. G. May, *Addiction and Grace* (San Francisco: Harper & Row, 1998).
8. M. Byrne, *A New North Wall Spirit* (Dublin: Elo Press, 1998), p. 8.
9. Ibid.
10. The names assigned are fictional.
11. This parallel was inspired by J. Langford, 'Ministry to Gen-X Catholics, Jesus Style', *America* (22 April 2000), pp. 6-10.
12. T. S. Eliot, 'The Social Function of Poetry', in *On Poetry and Poets* (New York: H. Wolf, 1961), 3-16 at 15.
13. Jean Vanier, *Becoming Human* (London: Darton, Longman & Todd, 1999).

Recommendations

From the fieldwork it is clear that there is a real need to help people working in the area of treatment/rehabilitation to access programmes and support spaces that would nourish their own spiritual development. To this end, the following recommendation has emerged:

> To resource a team of three people to work
> creatively in the area of spirituality and addiction.

It is recognised that this team would need to carry some degree of credibility – both for those working in the treatment/rehabilitation area and for those who would be the primary funders of the team's work. It was also recognised that there would firstly be a need to find a suitable person to spearhead this team, who would then be able to co-opt two other team members with complementary skills.

The team will endeavour to:

- Promote a theoretical understanding of the place of spirituality in the response to street drug culture.
- Create an awareness and facilitate the implementation of the Bishops' Policy Document 1997, *Breaking the Silence,* and the Bishops' Policy Document 1998, *Tackling Drug Problems Together.*
- Facilitate ongoing conversations with those interviewed who are working in the area of addiction and who expressed a wish to further engage with the issue.
- Provide and promote creative rituals.
- Develop and deliver explicit spiritual programmes for those working with and those affected by addiction.
- Train and empower others to do the same.
- Research into the links between spirituality and addiction.
- Network and link with international trends and practices.
- Document and evaluate work.

We feel that, as those afflicted by drug addiction are frequently the poorest and most hard-pressed in our country, they well warrant a serious and generous response.

Response to the Short Questionnaire

Of the 78 questionnaires that were sent out, there were 39 responses.

1.   Does your centre have an explicit spirituality component on its programme?

      YES: 14   NO: 25

2.   *Of the 14 who responded Yes:*
      8 identified the 12-step programme
      2 were from Cuan Mhuire centres
      3 were centres who had chaplains
      1 facilitated bereavement rituals.

3.   Does your centre have elements on its programme which you consider, implicitly, to be nourishing of your clients' spirits?

      YES: 31   NO: 8

4.   *Of the 31 who responded Yes:*
      9 identified elements of the 12-steps or use of serenity prayer, etc.
      14 identified counselling and working from a base of humanistic-integrative philosophy
      7 identified meditation, yoga, reiki and alternative therapies
      8 identified fellowship
      7 identified Christian prayer services or liturgies
      2 identified lectures that were given
      4 identified the atmosphere/spirit of the centre
      2 identified bereavement rituals
      2 identified art
      2 identified closeness to nature.

      Of the 8 who responded No:
      1 was from a help-line and offered no programmes
      1 was from a centre offering only treatment
      3 were from counsellors working in the addiction services.

5.   Would you be interested in further conversations with people who are reflecting on the relationship between spirituality and addiction?

       YES: 32   NO: 7

These 32 have all given their addresses for further communication.

Only three of those who responded wished to remain anonymous.

Conclusions
In general, there appear to be two dominant pathways to accessing explicit spirituality components in treatment or rehabilitation centres.

•   Centres that were set up by a dynamic founder whose own belief in spirituality was put centre stage and was subsequently accepted by the participants as part and parcel of the rehabilitation programme being offered in the centre.

•   Those centres that promote the 12-step programme as the pathway to recovery.

Both of these systems have permission from their participants to treat spirituality in an explicit and even central way. The dilemma is how to introduce or promote an attending to the spirit in centres that have no explicit spiritual component.

    Of the 39 centres that responded to the questionnaire, 32 indicated they would like to be part of further conversations on the topic. Most of these were then contacted by telephone or in person in order to clarify what respondents believed would be useful to them in bringing the issue further.

    Two others, who had since heard about the questionnaire, have also asked to be part of further conversations.

    There are many Christians from a 'Born Again' perspective who engage significantly with people suffering from addiction. This is an area that merits further exploration.